Public Health Mini-Guide
Diabetes

Josie Evans
Reader in Public Health, School of Health Sciences, University of Stirling, UK

Angela Scriven
Formerly Reader in Health Promotion, Brunel University, London, UK

Series editor
Angela Scriven

CHURCHILL
LIVINGSTONE

ELSEVIER

Edinburgh London New York Oxford Philadelphia St Louis Sydney Toronto 2016

CHURCHILL
LIVINGSTONE
ELSEVIER

ISBN 9780702046377
e_ISBN 9780702047145

British Library Cataloguing in Publication Data
A catalogue record for this book is available from the British Library

Library of Congress Cataloging in Publication Data
A catalog record for this book is available from the Library of Congress

Notices

Knowledge and best practice in this field are constantly changing. As new research and experience broaden our understanding, changes in research methods, professional practices, or medical treatment may become necessary.

Practitioners and researchers must always rely on their own experience and knowledge in evaluating and using any information, methods, compounds, or experiments described herein. In using such information or methods they should be mindful of their own safety and the safety of others, including parties for whom they have a professional responsibility.

With respect to any drug or pharmaceutical products identified, readers are advised to check the most current information provided (i) on procedures featured or (ii) by the manufacturer of each product to be administered, to verify the recommended dose or formula, the method and duration of administration, and contraindications. It is the responsibility of practitioners, relying on their own experience and knowledge of their patients, to make diagnoses, to determine dosages and the best treatment for each individual patient, and to take all appropriate safety precautions.

To the fullest extent of the law, neither the Publisher nor the authors, contributors, or editors assume any liability for any injury and/or damage to persons or property as a matter of products liability, negligence or otherwise, or from any use or operation of any methods, products, instructions, or ideas contained in the material herein.

ELSEVIER your source for books,
journals and multimedia
in the health sciences

www.elsevierhealth.com

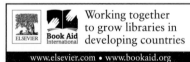

Working together
to grow libraries in
developing countries

www.elsevier.com • www.bookaid.org

The
Publisher's
policy is to use
**paper manufactured
from sustainable forests**

Printed in China

Contents

Titles in the Public Health Mini-Guides *series:*

Obesity
Nick Townsend, Angela Scriven
ISBN 9780702046346

Alcohol Misuse
Ken Barrie, Angela Scriven
ISBN 9780702046384

Diabetes
Josie Evans, Angela Scriven
ISBN 9780702046377

Series preface

The UK government highlighted in the Foreword to its strategy for public health in England, the *Healthy Lives, Healthy People* White Paper (The Stationery Office, 2010), some of the public health challenges that are facing those working to improve public health: 'Britain is now the most obese nation in Europe. We have among the worst rates of sexually transmitted infections recorded, a relatively large population of problem drug users and rising levels of harm from alcohol. Smoking alone claims over 80,000 lives in every year. Experts estimate that tackling poor mental health could reduce our overall disease burden by nearly a quarter. Health inequalities between rich and poor have been getting progressively worse'.

The public health targets are clear both in the White Paper and in *Our Health and Wellbeing Today* (Department of Health, 2010), published to accompany the White Paper, with the targets being supplemented by further policy drivers for mental health, tobacco control, obesity, sexual health and the wider determinants. The proposals and identified priorities in the White Paper apply to England, but they are of equal concern in the Devolved Administrations and globally, as evidenced in World Health Organization reports (www.who.int/whr/en/index. html). The *Public Health Mini-Guides* series covers some of the key health targets identified by the UK government and the WHO. The *Mini-Guides* highlight, in a concise, easily accessible manner, what the problems are and the range of potential solutions available to those professionals with a responsibility to promote health.

What the *Public Health Mini-Guides* provide

The *Mini-Guides* are written to provide up-to-date, evidence-based information in a convenient pocket-sized format, on a range of current key public health topics. They will support the work of health and social care practitioners and students on courses related to public health and health promotion.

Each volume provides an objective and balanced introduction to an overview of the epidemiological, scientific and other factors relating to public health. The *Mini-Guides* are structured to provide easy access to information. The first chapters cover background information needed to quickly understand the issue, including the epidemiology, demography and physiology. The later chapters examine examples of public health action to address the issue, covering health promotion intervention, legislative and other measures. The *Mini-Guides* are designed to be essential reference texts for students, practitioners and researchers with a professional interest in public health and health promotion.

Uxbridge, 2015

Angela Scriven

References

Department of Health. Our health and wellbeing today. London: Department of Health; 2010.
The Stationery Office. Healthy lives, healthy people. White paper, 2010.

Introduction

It is estimated that 380 million people in the world will have diabetes by the year 2025, with an annual global cost of 561 billion ID (international dollars). The World Health Organization has predicted that diabetes will become the seventh-leading cause of death worldwide by 2030. Against a backdrop of increasing incidence and prevalence, diabetes is now a worldwide public health concern and is being referred to as the 'global epidemic of diabetes', the 'silent epidemic' and the 'diabetes time bomb'.

Diabetes is a metabolic disorder with a long history, with the earliest description made by Aretaeus of Cappadocia in AD 100, although reference was made to possible symptoms of diabetes in an Egyptian papyrus dating back to 1550 BC. It was Indian physicians in the fifth and sixth centuries who first alluded to two different forms of diabetes. In Europe by the seventeenth century, taste-testing of the urine for sweetness was the main approach to clinical diagnosis of diabetes, and the presence of sugars in the urine, although established by increasingly more objective methods, remained the keystone to diabetes diagnosis until relatively recently.

Indeed, chronic hyperglycaemia (excess levels of glucose in the blood) is one of the defining features of diabetes, and results from an inability to regulate blood glucose levels. This is due to problems in either insulin secretion or insulin action. In addition to acute metabolic complications of diabetes (including diabetic ketoacidosis and hypoglycaemia), diabetes is associated with microvascular damage to the eyes, nerves and kidneys (retinopathy, neuropathy and nephropathy), an increased risk of macrovascular complications (ischaemic heart disease, stroke and peripheral vascular disease), lowered life expectancy and reduced quality of life.

The increasing incidence of diabetes, the heavy burden of morbidity and mortality associated with diabetes, and its spiralling health care costs underpin the importance of a public health approach to the prevention and management of diabetes. The following chapters explore in more detail how public health practice might address some of these issues.

World Health Organization 10 facts about diabetes

1. There is an emerging global epidemic of diabetes that can be traced back to rapid increases in overweight, obesity and physical inactivity.
2. Total deaths from diabetes are projected to rise by more than 50% in the next 10 years. Most notably, they are projected to increase by over 80% in upper-middle income countries.
3. Type 1 diabetes is characterised by a lack of insulin production and type 2 diabetes results from the body's ineffective use of insulin.
4. Type 2 diabetes is much more common than type 1 diabetes, and accounts for around 90% of all diabetes worldwide.
5. Reports of type 2 diabetes in children – previously rare – have increased worldwide. In some countries, it accounts for almost half of newly diagnosed cases in children and adolescents.
6. A third type of diabetes is gestational diabetes. This type is characterised by hyperglycaemia, or raised blood sugar, which is first recognised during pregnancy.
7. In 2005, 1.1 million people died from diabetes. The full impact is much larger, because although people may live for years with diabetes, their cause of death is often recorded as heart disease or kidney failure.
8. 80% of diabetes deaths are now occurring in low- and middle-income countries.
9. Lack of awareness about diabetes, combined with insufficient access to health services, can lead to complications such as blindness, amputation and kidney failure.
10. Diabetes can be prevented. Thirty minutes of moderate-intensity physical activity on most days and a healthy diet can drastically reduce the risk of developing type 2 diabetes.

These facts are reproduced verbatim from the World Health Organization website: http://www.who.int/features/factfiles/diabetes/10_en.html

1 Definitions and epidemiology of diabetes

Diabetes mellitus is a chronic disease characterised by hyperglycaemia: excessive levels of glucose in the blood. The condition results from insulin deficiency or insulin resistance. Insulin is the hormone produced by the pancreas that is essential for regulating carbohydrate and fat metabolism in the body (Box 1.1).

History of diabetes

Diabetes has a long history, with the earliest description made by Aretaeus of Cappadocia in AD 100, when he referred to it as 'the mysterious sickness'. He is credited with coining the term *diabetes*, derived from a Greek word meaning siphon and referring to excessive urination. However, there is possible reference to symptoms of diabetes in an Egyptian papyrus dating back to 1550 BC. Indian physicians in the fifth and sixth centuries first alluded to two different forms of diabetes, with one form associated with older age and being overweight, and one associated with younger age. This latter form was rapidly fatal.

By the seventeenth century in Europe it was recognised that diabetes was associated with sweetness of the urine, and taste-testing the urine was the main approach to clinical diagnosis. Indeed, the presence of sugars in the urine, although established by increasingly more objective methods, has remained the keystone to diabetes diagnosis until relatively recently. *Mellitus* comes from the Latin word meaning sweet like honey, and the term *diabetes mellitus* was first used at the turn of the eighteenth century. However, until the twentieth century the prognosis for people diagnosed with diabetes was poor. The life expectancy of children after they were diagnosed with diabetes was less than a year. The lives of people with diabetes could be prolonged slightly by prescribing them very low calorie diets but this kept them in a state of near starvation.

It was the discovery of insulin in 1921 that proved to be a turning

---

Box 1.1 Carbohydrate metabolism and the action of insulin

Levels of glucose in the blood are controlled by a complex interaction between the gastrointestinal system, the pancreas and the liver. During digestion, after food has been ingested, carbohydrates are broken down into glucose molecules. Glucose is then absorbed into the blood, elevating blood glucose levels. This triggers the secretion of insulin from the beta cells of the pancreas. Insulin binds to specific cellular receptors, where it can facilitate entry of glucose into the cells of the body to be used for energy. Increased insulin secretion from the pancreas and the use of glucose by the cells of the body then results in a lowering of blood glucose levels and decreased subsequent insulin secretion.

However, if there are problems with insulin production and secretion, these dynamics can change. If insulin production is insufficient or if insulin is not used properly by the cells of the body, glucose cannot enter cells efficiently, and blood glucose levels can become too high (hyperglycaemia). Conversely, if there is an increase in insulin secretion, blood glucose levels can become too low as excessive amounts of glucose enter cells (hypoglycaemia).

The amount of glucose in the blood may exceed the amount of glucose required by cells for energy. Excess glucose is then stored in the liver as glycogen, which can be converted back to glucose when required and used to increase blood glucose levels. The liver can also produce glucose from fat and proteins.

Box 1.2 Pathophysiology of type 1 and type 2 diabetes

The underlying pathophysiology in type 1 diabetes is an autoimmune destruction of pancreatic beta cells. An individual with type 1 diabetes can no longer produce insulin and therefore has a lifelong requirement for insulin treatment.

In contrast, there is no beta cell destruction in type 2 diabetes. Type 2 diabetes is characterised by peripheral resistance to insulin, increased glucose production by the liver and altered insulin secretion. Increased tissue resistance to insulin generally occurs first. The pancreas produces insulin, but resistance to insulin prevents its effective use by the cells of the body. Therefore glucose cannot enter cells and accumulates in the blood, resulting in hyperglycaemia. These high blood glucose levels can then trigger an increase in insulin production by the pancreas, with many people with type 2 diabetes having excessive insulin production (hyperinsulinaemia) – although this is a symptom not a cause of diabetes. People with type 2 diabetes do not necessarily require treatment with insulin but can attempt to control their blood glucose levels using oral hypoglycaemic therapies or by lifestyle management.

point in diabetes treatment and care. The experiments of Dr Frederick Banting, with medical student Charles Best, showed that the high blood sugars of diabetic dogs could be lowered by injecting them with material extracted from the islets of Langerhans of the pancreas. The material extracted was named insulin, after the Latin word for 'island'. Work then proceeded on purification of the insulin that had been discovered. In January 1922, Leonard Thompson, a 14-year-old boy dying from diabetes in Toronto, Canada, was the first patient to be injected with exogenous insulin. He lived for another 13 years, eventually dying from pneumonia. The Nobel Prize was awarded to Frederick Banting and Professor John JR McLeod of the University of Toronto for this breakthrough, although they shared their winnings with Charles Best and James Bertram Collip, the chemist who had assisted with the purification process. Eli Lilly, a US pharmaceutical company, was granted manufacturing rights to insulin, and they were able to produce it on a large scale.

Since its discovery, the lives of millions of people with diabetes have been saved by insulin. But diabetes care in the twentieth century is characterised by other landmark developments. Pork and beef insulin were first manufactured in the 1930s, and following this

has come the production of longer-acting preparations of insulin. The oral hypoglycaemic agents known as sulfonylureas were discovered in the 1950s. Urine test strips to measure the levels of glucose in the urine were introduced in the 1960s. In 1961, single-use syringes were made available to patients, replacing the glass syringes that needed to be repeatedly boiled and sterilised. The first blood glucose meter was used in 1969. The first insulin pumps were introduced at the end of the 1970s, although the initial prototypes were heavy and bulky. The first production of human insulin from genetically modified bacteria occurred in 1982. The use of metformin was approved in 1995.

Although Dr Roger Hinsworth described two different types of diabetes in 1935, diabetes has a multifactorial aetiology, and several different types are now recognised. The three most common are type 1 diabetes, type 2 diabetes and gestational diabetes, defined as follows (Boxes 1.2–1.4).

Definitions

Type 1 diabetes accounts for around 10% of all cases of diabetes. It is a progressive autoimmune disease, in which insulin-producing beta cells in the pancreas are gradually destroyed, resulting in insulin deficiency.

Box 1.3 Diagnostic criteria for diabetes

Plasma glucose measurements are used to diagnosis diabetes. The World Health Organization first published technical guidelines for the diagnosis and classification of diabetes in 1965, and since then they have been reviewed and updated several times. There is ongoing debate on whether diabetes should be regarded as a discrete clinical entity or the upper end of a continuous distribution. The currently recommended WHO/IDF guidelines date from 2006.

Diagnostic criteria for diabetes are either a fasting plasma glucose ≥ 7.0 mmol/L or a 2-h plasma glucose ≥ 11.1 mmol/L (oral glucose tolerance test). Diagnostic criteria for IGT are a fasting plasma glucose <7.0 mmol/L and a 2-h plasma glucose of 7.8–11.0 mmol/L. The diagnostic criterion for IFG is a fasting plasma glucose of 6.1–6.9 mmol/L. It is recommended that a 2-h plasma glucose be used to exclude IGT.

Source: WHO/IDF Consultation Group (2006).

Box 1.4 Use of haemoglobin A1c (HbA1c) in the diagnosis of diabetes

In a later addendum to their 2006 report, the World Health Organization reported on evidence for the use of glycosylated haemoglobin (HbA1c) as a test for diabetes. They make the following recommendations:

- HbA1c can be used as a diagnostic test for diabetes providing that stringent quality assurance tests are in place and assays are standardised to criteria aligned to the international reference values and that there are no conditions present that preclude the accurate measurement of HbA1c.
- An HbA1c of 6.5% is recommended as the cut point for diagnosing diabetes. A value of less than 6.5% does not exclude diabetes.

Although glucose testing is not routinely recommended in people with HbA1c of less than 6.5% (48 mmol/mol), it is advisable for patients with symptoms of diabetes or who are clinically at very high risk of diabetes.

Source: World Health Organization (2011).

Previously called juvenile-onset diabetes or insulin-dependent diabetes, patients are usually diagnosed during childhood or adolescence and require lifelong treatment with insulin (World Health Organization, 1999).

Type 2 diabetes is the most common form of diabetes and is the result of abnormalities in insulin secretion, together with insulin resistance, when the insulin that is produced by the body is not effective. Previously known as adult-onset diabetes or non-insulin-dependent diabetes, it is associated with obesity and a sedentary lifestyle, usually presents over the age of 40 years

Table 1.1 Diagnostic criteria for diabetes mellitus and states of intermediate hyperglycaemia

FASTING PLASMA GLUCOSE (mmol/L)	2-h PLASMA GLUCOSE (mmol/L)		
	<7.8	7.8–11.0	≥11.1
≥7.0	Diabetes	Diabetes	Diabetes
6.1–6.9	Impaired fasting glucose	Impaired glucose tolerance	Diabetes
≤6.0	Normoglycaemia	Impaired glucose tolerance	Diabetes

Source: WHO/IDF Consultation Group (2006).

and does not necessarily require treatment with insulin (World Health Organization, 1999).

Gestational diabetes is defined as glucose intolerance first diagnosed during pregnancy. Although most women return to normal glucose tolerance after delivery, they are at high risk of developing type 2 diabetes in later life (American Diabetes Association, 2003a).

Other, less common, forms of diabetes include various forms of maturity-onset diabetes of the young, where there is mutation in a single gene, secondary diabetes associated with conditions such as chronic pancreatitis and cystic fibrosis, diabetes associated with other genetic syndromes, and drug- or toxin-induced diabetes (Libman et al., 2011).

Impaired glucose tolerance (IGT) and impaired fasting glucose (IFG) represent two other states of intermediate hyperglycaemia that are not normal, but

neither are they diagnostic of diabetes (see Table 1.1 for further information). The term prediabetes is also used to refer to intermediate hyperglycaemia. IGT and IFG are associated, either alone or in combination, with varying increased risks of diabetes.

Epidemiology of diabetes

Incidence and prevalence are commonly used measures of disease frequency in a population. The incidence of a disease is the number of new cases arising in the population during a defined period of time. The prevalence of a disease refers to the total number of existing cases of disease in the population.

Incidence and prevalence of type 1 diabetes

Over 70,000 children in the world develop type 1 diabetes every year, with the majority of cases arising in young people under the age of 15 years. In the

United Kingdom, around 2000 children are diagnosed with type 1 diabetes annually. The incidence of type 1 diabetes internationally varies markedly, but the highest incidence appears to occur in Caucasian or European populations. The DIAMOND study used standardised criteria to determine the age-standardised incidence of type 1 diabetes in 50 countries between 1990 and 1994 and found that it ranged from 0.1/100,000 per year in China and Venezuela to >36/100,000 per year in the United Kingdom and Finland (DIAMOND Project Group, 2006). The EURODIAB study noted a high incidence rate in Finland, as well as an overall increase in incidence over the time period, particularly in children aged 0–4 years (EURODIAB ACE Study Group, 2000). The incidence of type 1 diabetes appears to be rising. It has been estimated that the average increase in incidence of type 1 diabetes was 3.0% per year in 27 countries between 1960 and 1996 (Onkamo et al., 2000) and 3.9% in 20 European countries between 1989 and 2003 (Patterson et al., 2009).

There are around 400,000 people with type 1 diabetes in the United Kingdom (overall prevalence of 0.6%), with approximately 1 in every 700–1000 children affected.

Incidence and prevalence of type 2 diabetes

The global increasing incidence of type 2 diabetes is now well recognised and has become a major public health concern. It is driven in part by the obesity epidemic and, coupled with the effects of ageing populations, is also causing a worldwide increase in diabetes prevalence.

The Framingham Heart Study identified a doubling in the incidence of type 2 diabetes among around 5000 adults in Framingham, MA, between the 1970s and the 1990s (Fox et al., 2006). Over a 10-year period in the United Kingdom, the incidence of type 2 diabetes increased from 2.60 to 4.31 cases per 1000 patient years (Masso Gonzalez et al., 2009). The increases are also evident in low- and middle-income countries, as these become more affluent and urbanised and populations go through lifestyle adaptations, including nutritional transition. For example, The Singapore Chinese Health Study carried out among more than 43,000 people found the incidence of type 2 diabetes to be over 9 per 1000 patient years between 1993 and 1998 (Odegaard et al., 2011). Although there have been few incidence studies carried out in the Middle East, a recent study in Iran estimated incidence to be as high as 10 per 1000 patient-years (Harati et al., 2009). The emerging burden of type 2 diabetes in African countries has also been well described (Mbanya et al., 2010).

According to the IDF Diabetes Atlas (International Diabetes Federation, 2013a), 382 million adults now have diabetes, compared with 171 million in

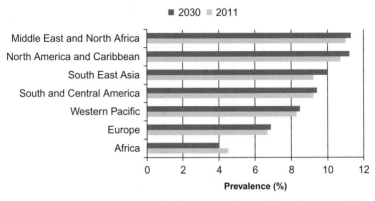

Fig. 1.1 *Estimated (2011) and projected (2030) prevalence of type 2 diabetes in seven world regions.*
Source: International Diabetes Federation (2011a).

2000 (Wild et al., 2004). This equates to over 8% of all adults. Although the prevalence in high-income countries is still higher than in countries with developing economies (see Fig. 1.1 for regional variations), these patterns are likely to change over the next few decades. Currently, 80% of all people with diabetes live in developing countries.

! Thinking point

Why do you think the prevalence of diabetes is projected to come down in Africa by 2030, but not in any other region?

In 2012, there were approximately 3,400,000 people with type 2 diabetes in the United Kingdom, giving an overall prevalence of around 5%, but this varies by region and population

group. Prevalence increases with age. For example, prevalence in England (including people with type 1 and type 2 diabetes) ranges from around 2% in people less than 35 years of age to over 15% in men over 65 years, and over 12% in women of this age (Diabetes UK, 2012a). In the Health Survey for England, doctor-diagnosed type 2 diabetes was at least twice as prevalent among Black Caribbean, Black African, Pakistani, Bangladeshi and Indian men and women (Health Survey for England, 2004). There is also a strong association between the prevalence of type 2 diabetes and socioeconomic status, as described in a study in Tayside, Scotland (Evans et al., 2000). This is also illustrated in Fig. 1.2, where the prevalence of type 2 diabetes in 2009/2010 was determined in the National Diabetes Audit for England

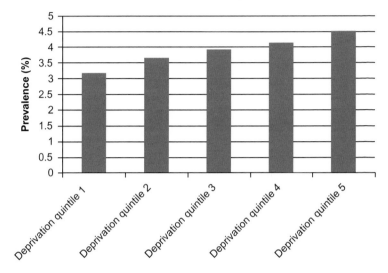

Fig. 1.2 *Prevalence of type 2 diabetes in England, 2009/2010, stratified by deprivation quintile (least deprived is quintile 1).*
Source: The NHS Information Centre (2011).

stratified by quintile of deprivation, clearly illustrating increasing prevalence with increasing deprivation (The NHS Information Centre, 2011).

Risk factors for type 1 diabetes

There are several modifiable and nonmodifiable risk factors for type 1 diabetes (Maahs et al., 2010). The risk of type 1 diabetes increases from birth and peaks between the ages of 10 and 14 years. On average, there appears to be little difference in risk between males and females; however, although no studies have reported a higher incidence among females, some studies have reported a higher incidence for males (DIAMOND Project Group, 2006).

All first-degree relatives (including parents) of an individual diagnosed with type 1 diabetes are also at increased risk of the disease. For example, their siblings have a risk of developing type 1 diabetes of between 1 in 10 and 1 in 30, their parents of 1 in 34 and their offspring of 1 in 20 (Gregory et al., 2010). This increased risk is present to a lesser extent in second- and third-degree relatives. This suggests that there is a strong genetic component to type 1 diabetes, with several specific genes identified that increase susceptibility to the disease (Wanatabe et al.,

2007). However, many genetic risk factors remain unknown. Despite this genetic element to type 1 diabetes, the proportion of people at high genetic risk who go on to develop type 1 diabetes is still relatively low. Furthermore, around 90% of newly diagnosed patients have no family history of the disease. This indicates that there are also likely to be important environmental risk factors.

Apart from the wide geographical differences in risk, which generally increase with increasing distance from the equator, a possible environmental risk factor is vitamin D levels at birth (which might explain differences in risk by month of birth), with vitamin D supplementation of the pregnant mother and infant associated with a reduced risk. Other possible diet-related risk factors include cow's milk, vitamin E deficiency and early introduction of cereals to the infant diet, although none are unequivocally confirmed. Infectious diseases are implicated in the onset of type 1 diabetes, with viral exposure and insufficient exposure to early infections (the so-called hygiene hypothesis) associated with increased risk. The seasonal variation in infections would also explain the confirmed seasonal variation in type 1 diabetes, with most cases occurring over the winter period.

Risk factors for type 2 diabetes

Mayer-Davis et al. (2011) argue that an ecologic approach is useful for an understanding of the risk of type 2 diabetes. Rather than tackling risk factors in isolation, this approach sees risk of disease emerging as a product of individuals interacting with their social, cultural and physical environments. Type 2 diabetes is a complex disease, and multiple risk factors have been identified, many of which may be overlapping and interrelated.

Nonmodifiable risk factors for type 2 diabetes

These include:

- Age
- Family history
- Genetic susceptibility
- Ethnic origin

Age Historically, type 2 diabetes was regarded as a disease of middle age, with most cases arising in people over the age of 40 years. However, there has been a worrying trend for increasing numbers of diagnoses in people younger than this, and even in children (Fagot-Campagna et al., 2001).

Family history This is an important risk factor and reflects both genetic and environmental origins. Having a parent with diabetes may increase the risk of diabetes up to sixfold, with the higher estimates where the parent is the mother (Harrison et al., 2003).

Genetic susceptibility Many gene variants confer susceptibility to type 2 diabetes (Wanatabe et al., 2007) but the effects are relatively modest, and genetic screening is not warranted.

Ethnic origin Self-identified race and ethnicity also appear to be risk factors for type 2 diabetes, with a particularly high incidence noted among people of South Asian, African, African-Caribbean and Middle Eastern descent. In the United Kingdom, the prevalence of type 2 diabetes is much higher in South Asian communities than in the general population; some reports suggest it is up to five times higher (Health Survey for England, 2004).

Modifiable risk factors for type 2 diabetes

These include:

- Overweight and obesity
- Low levels of physical activity

Overweight and obesity The most important modifiable risk factor for type 2 diabetes is excess body fat. Overall obesity and central obesity (as measured by waist-to-hip ratio or waist circumference) are strong, independent predictors of diabetes. With the prevalence of obesity estimated at over one-quarter in many high-income countries, overweight and obesity are implicated in 60% of all cases of diabetes (Yach et al., 2006). Obesity leads to the development of insulin resistance and to dysfunction of the insulin-secreting beta cells in the pancreas, both of which are strong independent risk factors for type 2 diabetes. Insulin resistance triples the risk for type 2 diabetes. Figs 1.3 and 1.4 illustrate the

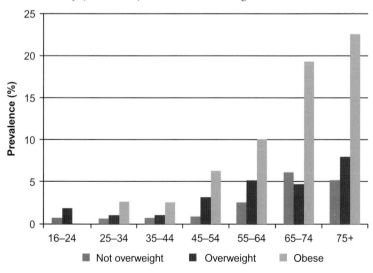

Fig. 1.3 *Prevalence of doctor-diagnosed diabetes among women in England, 2006, by age and BMI status.*
Source: The Information Centre (2008).

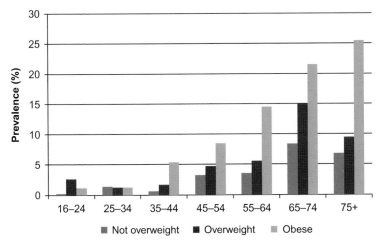

Fig. 1.4 *Prevalence of doctor-diagnosed diabetes among men in England, 2006, by age and BMI status.*
Source: The Information Centre (2008).

relationship between prevalence of diabetes and overweight and obesity among males and females respectively in England.

Weight management plays an essential role in reducing the risk of type 2 diabetes. In terms of diet, there needs to be an emphasis on reduced total energy intake and also reduced intake of foods with high levels of fats, sugars and alcohol. Other dietary habits may also be important, independent of weight status. Diets characterised by high intake of red and processed meats, sweets, fried foods and refined grains may increase the risk of diabetes compared with diets with higher intake of fruit, vegetables, fish, poultry and whole grain. Similarly, reduced intake of

fats (especially saturated fats), increased intake of whole grains and dietary fibre, increased intake of low-fat dairy products, and increased consumption of nuts, have all been associated with a reduced risk of diabetes (see Chapter 6 for public health interventions relating to reducing the risk of type 2 diabetes).

Low levels of physical activity With high proportions of the populations of high-income countries not meeting minimum physical activity recommendations for health, a sedentary lifestyle is another important modifiable risk factor for type 2 diabetes. The effects of physical activity on reducing the risk of type 2 diabetes arise not only through weight management, but also through the favourable effects that physical activity confers on insulin sensitivity, glycaemic control, blood pressure, lipid profile, fibrinolysis, endothelial function and inflammatory defence systems.

! Thinking point

Consider the prevalence rates for men and women in England that are outlined in Figs 1.2 and 1.3. Why do you think that overweight and obesity appear to become greater risk factors for developing diabetes over the age of 35?

The metabolic syndrome The presence of the metabolic syndrome is a recognised risk factor for type 2 diabetes, conferring at least a fivefold increased risk of developing the disease. The International Diabetes Federation states that for a person to be defined as having the metabolic syndrome, they must have central obesity, together with at least two of the following four risk factors: raised triglycerides, reduced HDL cholesterol, raised blood pressure and raised fasting plasma glucose (International Diabetes Federation, 2006). Up to one-quarter of the world's population is thought to have the metabolic syndrome.

Other suggested risk factors for type 2 diabetes include smoking, dysfunctional sleep patterns and depression, although the direction of causality may be uncertain, and the associations may be confounded by other known risk factors (such as obesity).

With increasing interest in a life course approach to risk, and drawing on Barker's (1999) fetal origins hypothesis, there are several risk factors from early life that increase the risk of type 2 diabetes. These include either small or large birth weight, exposure to diabetes in utero (with the mother having diabetes or gestational diabetes during pregnancy) and not being breastfed in early life.

A well-established risk factor for type 2 diabetes is low socioeconomic position. Although this association may be explained by many of the risk factors mentioned earlier, it illustrates the importance of taking an ecologic approach to the prevention of type 2 diabetes, where individual behavioural risk factors, such as obesity or diet, cannot be addressed without relating to the individual's social and cultural environment. This will be explored further in Chapter 6.

Gestational diabetes

Gestational diabetes is defined as glucose intolerance first diagnosed during pregnancy, and it affects around 5–7% of all pregnancies worldwide (American Diabetes Association, 2003b). The risk increases with each successive pregnancy, so the prevalence is higher in multiparous women (up to 13%). The prevalence appears to be increasing, with Ferrara (2007) presenting evidence from six studies, four from the United States and two from Australia, all of which documented such an increase over the last few decades. However, one of the methodological challenges in assessing the prevalence of gestational diabetes is that it may not be possible to distinguish between underlying diabetes that existed prior to the pregnancy and gestational diabetes itself. The increasing prevalence is probably due to the trend towards older maternal age and the epidemic of obesity (Ferrara, 2007).

Risk factors for gestational diabetes

These include:

- Being overweight before pregnancy (BMI >30 kg/m^2)
- Older maternal age
- Having a first-degree relative with diabetes
- Previous glucose intolerance
- Previous macrosomia (baby with birth weight >4.5 kg)
- Polycystic ovarian syndrome
- Being from an ethnic group with high prevalence of gestational diabetes, including South Asian, Black Caribbean and Middle Eastern

Women with a history of gestational diabetes have a high risk of developing type 2 diabetes later in life, and whether gestational diabetes should even be regarded as a separate disease entity has been questioned.

The frequency of gestational diabetes is related to the frequency of type 2 diabetes in the underlying population. Gestational diabetes is more common in ethnic minority groups. For example, in the United States, Native Americans, Asians, Hispanics and African-American women have a higher risk than non-Hispanic white women; gestational diabetes is also more common among Asian women in Europe compared to European women.

Prediabetes/impaired glucose regulation

IFG and IGT, collectively known as impaired glucose regulation (IGR) or prediabetes, are designations used for people whose blood glucose levels are above the normal range, but not high enough to be diagnostic of diabetes. IFG and IGT can occur separately or in combination, but it is recommended that people with IFG also be tested for IGT (see Table 1.1). People with IGR have a 5- to 15-fold increased risk of type 2 diabetes, with 40–50% of all patients with an IGT diagnosis developing type 2 diabetes within 10 years and high 1-year progression rates from IGT to type 2 diabetes also reported (Nathan et al., 2007). However, IGR is asymptomatic and can remain undiagnosed for many years.

Among all adults, the prevalence of IGR is likely to be around 15%. A study using data from 13 European countries using WHO 1999 diagnostic criteria for diagnosis of diabetes suggested that the prevalence of IGT, but not IFG, increased with age, and that the overall prevalence of IGR was less than 15% in people under the age of 60 years, but between 15% and 30% in people older than this (The DECODE Study Group, 2003). The diagnosis of IGR provides an important opportunity for intervention to prevent or delay progression to diabetes.

Undiagnosed diabetes

The onset of type 2 diabetes can occur several years before clinical diagnosis; the International Diabetes Federation (2013) estimates that 46% of all people with diabetes worldwide have not yet been diagnosed, with the majority of them living in low- and middle-income countries. There is more chance of preventing long-term complications of diabetes with earlier detection and treatment, so many people living with undiagnosed diabetes will already have developed complications of diabetes when they are finally diagnosed. For example, a study of 1077 newly diagnosed patients in the United Kingdom in 1990–1992, indicated that only 360 (33%) were free from diabetic complications at diagnosis (Ruigomez and Garcia-Rodriguez, 1998). In the United Kingdom Prospective Diabetes Study (UK Prospective Diabetes Study Group, 1990), around one-quarter of newly diagnosed patients had already developed complications.

It is possible to estimate the prevalence of undiagnosed diabetes when population-based surveys are undertaken and people are found to have diabetes who have not previously been diagnosed, even though they may have had diabetes for some length of time. The International Diabetes Federation has summarised results from 81 population-based surveys across the world that quantified the proportion of the overall number of cases of

diabetes in the population (identified in the surveys) that had previously been diagnosed (International Diabetes Federation, 2006b). These are shown in Table 1.2. Overall, only around one-half of all people with diabetes were known cases of diabetes. In general, the lowest percentages were seen in developing countries, suggesting a high prevalence of undiagnosed diabetes in the population, and the highest percentages were from developed countries, suggesting a lower prevalence. In Tanzania, rural India, Nepal, Tonga and China only 20–25% of all people with diabetes had been previously diagnosed.

The number of people in the United Kingdom with undiagnosed diabetes has been estimated to be over 1 million. The equivalent number in the United States is estimated to be 8.1 million (National Diabetes Statistics Report, 2014).

The economic burden of diabetes

The cost of managing diabetes places a huge burden on global health services. Zhang et al. (2010) estimated that 12% of global health expenditure was for diabetes in 2010. They modelled the global health expenditure in 193 countries among adults aged 20–79 years using age- and sex-specific ratios of expenditure for people with and without diabetes. Overall, they estimated that 379 billion US dollars (USD) were spent on diabetes in 2010 and forecast this to increase to 490 billion USD by 2030.

Table 1.2 Summary of results of 82 studies estimating known cases of diabetes as a proportion of total cases of diabetes

WORLD REGION	NUMBER OF STUDIES INCLUDED	KNOWN CASES OF DIABETES AS PROPORTION OF TOTAL CASES OF DIABETES (%)	
		MEAN	MEDIAN
Africa	6	33	26
Eastern Mediterranean and Middle East	18	57	57
Europe	25	53	51
North America	4	71	76
South and Central America	5	58	55
South East Asia	7	38	32
Western Pacific	17	46	50

Source: International Diabetes Federation (2006b).

The proportion of a country's health expenditure spent on diabetes varies from 2% to 41%, although this figure depends on the prevalence of diabetes in the country. Fig. 1.5 shows this proportion for seven international regions. There is also huge variation in the expenditure per person with diabetes, ranging from less than 10 USD to over 7000 USD, as presented in Fig. 1.6, again for the seven regions.

The costs estimated by Zhang et al. (2010) were direct costs, that is, those directly incurred by health services for managing and treating diabetes. The International Diabetes Federation estimates that, in industrialised countries, around quarter of expenditures on diabetes is for blood glucose control, around one-quarter for the treatment of long-term complications of diabetes and the remaining half for additional general medical care (including prevention of diabetic complications). In contrast, in middle-income countries, a higher proportion of expenditure is for blood glucose control (around half), with the remaining proportion spent on complications and general medical care.

However, there are also indirect costs attributable to diabetes. These refer to other costs borne by society such as mortality, sickness, loss of productivity among people at work (presenteeism) and informal care. For example, the American Diabetes Association estimated that, in 2002, the US economy lost 3290 USD per person with diabetes (an overall total of 39.8 billion USD), in addition to over 7000 USD of direct health care expenditures.

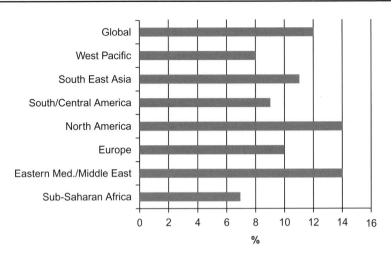

Fig. 1.5 *Proportion of health expenditure on diabetes as a proportion of total health expenditure for countries within seven international regions.*
Source: Zhang et al. (2010).

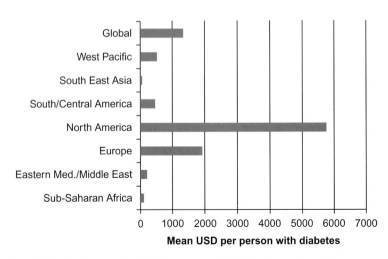

Fig. 1.6 *Mean health expenditure (USD) per person with diabetes for countries within seven international regions.*
Source: Zhang et al. (2010).

Hex et al. (2012) carried out a detailed examination of direct and indirect costs attributable to diabetes in the United Kingdom for 2010/2011. They estimated the annual costs of diabetes in the United Kingdom to be £23.7 billion. This is £1.9 billion for type 1 diabetes (£1 billion direct and £0.9 billion indirect costs) and £23.8 billion for type 2 diabetes (£8.8 billion direct and £13 billion indirect costs). Tables 1.3 and 1.4 break down these costs in detail.

Table 1.3 Direct costs of diabetes in the UK, 2010/2011 (£ millions)

	TYPE 1 DIABETES	TYPE 2 DIABETES
Screening and testing		
Diagnosis	1.44	8.17
Retinopathy screening	0.27	2.41
Treatment and management		
Primary care	98.08	950.71
Prescriptions	155.48	701.79
Insulin pumps	19.94	0.14
Continuous glucose monitoring	0.57	–
Influenza immunisation	5.75	49.21
Medical exemption	5.33	48.01
Education programmes	4.03	0.77
Smoking cessation programmes	0.64	5.52
Complications		
Hypoglycaemia (moderate)	19.19	22.61
Hypoglycaemia (severe)	13.94	16.43
Dyslipidaemia	2.75	24.72
Neuropathy	43.00	266.63
Erectile dysfunction	1.85	11.47
Ketoacidosis	15.96	–
Hyperglycaemia	5.64	50.80
Ischaemic heart disease	50.97	458.69
Myocardial infarction	29.27	573.80
Heart failure	30.82	277.34
Stroke	13.93	274.00
Kidney failure	135.06	379.00
Other renal costs	51.56	374.84
Retinopathy	5.77	51.97

Continued

Table 1.3 Direct costs of diabetes in the UK, 2010/2011 (£ millions)—cont'd

	TYPE 1 DIABETES	TYPE 2 DIABETES
Foot ulcers and amputation	111.59	874.00
Depression	3.32	29.89
Gestational diabetes	–	4.29
Other cardiovascular disease	165.49	1654.86
Diabetic medicine outpatients	1.63	16.34
Excess inpatient days	17.36	1822.83

Source: Hex et al. (2012).

Table 1.4 Indirect costs of diabetes in the UK, 2010/2011 (£ millions)

	TYPE 1 DIABETES	TYPE 2 DIABETES
Mortality	560.34	4203.54
Sickness absence	94.56	851.02
Presenteeism	91.05	2943.81
Informal care	153.29	4956.42

Source: Hex et al. (2012).

 Summary points

- Diabetes mellitus is a chronic disease characterised by hyperglycaemia (excessive levels of glucose in the blood) and is caused by an inability to regulate blood glucose levels. This is due to problems in insulin secretion or insulin action.
- There are several different types of diabetes, and it has a multifactorial aetiology. The three most common types are type 1 diabetes, type 2 diabetes and gestational diabetes.
- Type 2 diabetes accounts for 85–90% of all cases of diabetes.
- The incidence and prevalence of type 2 diabetes is increasing rapidly, with prevalence of around 8% for all adults worldwide. The prevalence of gestational diabetes is also increasing.
- The incidence of type 1 diabetes is increasing, particularly in very young children.
- These trends are evident in the United Kingdom, where there are around 400,000 and 3,400,000 people with type 1 and type 2 diabetes respectively, costing around £23.7 billion per year (£9.8 billion in direct costs, £23.7 billion in indirect costs).

Summary points—cont'd

- The most important modifiable risk factor for type 2 diabetes and gestational diabetes is excess body fat, with the worldwide increase in overweight and obesity fuelling a diabetes epidemic.
- Around 15% of adults have IGR, putting them at up to 15 times the risk of developing type 2 diabetes.
- Undiagnosed diabetes is a significant problem, with nearly half of all people with diabetes not yet diagnosed.
- Around 12% of health expenditure globally is for diabetes.

Web pages and resources

The following organisations campaign to raise awareness of diabetes, promote appropriate diabetes care and prevention and support research for finding a cure.

Diabetes UK. www.diabetes.org.uk.

A leading UK charity.

American Diabetes Association. www.diabetes.org.

A leading US charity.

International Diabetes Federation. www.idf.org.

A global alliance of around 200 diabetes associations in more than 160 countries.

Facts and figures

www.idf.org/diabetesatlas

This atlas is an authoritative source of evidence on the burden of diabetes worldwide.

www.who.int/diabetes/en

This is the home page of the WHO Diabetes programme, providing access to a range of data sources and publications, including:

World Health Organization Diabetes Programme. Facts and figures about diabetes. www.who.int/diabetes/facts/world-figures

Here you can find figures on current and projected prevalence of diabetes by region and country.

Diabetes UK. Diabetes: Facts and Stats. https://www.diabetes.org.uk/Documents/About%20Us/Statistics/Diabetes-key-stats-guidelines-April2014.pdf

This report from Diabetes UK provides the most up-to-date figures on the burden of diabetes in the United Kingdom.

2014 National Diabetes Statistics Report. http://www.cdc.gov/diabetes/data/statistics/2014statisticsreport.html

Here, the Centers for Disease Control and Prevention provide up-to-date data and statistics on diabetes and its burden in the United States.

Further reading

Craig ME, Hattersley A, Donaghue KC. Definition, epidemiology and classification of diabetes in children and adolescents. Pediatr Diabetes 2009;10(Suppl. 12):3–12.

As the title implies, this article offers a very detailed overview of the epidemiology and classification of diabetes in children and adolescents. This is an important paper for those working with these groups.

Massó González EL, Johnasson S, Wallender M-A, Gracia-Rodriguez LA. Trends in the prevalence and incidence of diabetes in the UK: 1996–2005. J Epidemiol Community Health 2009;63:332–6.

The incidence and prevalence of type 1 and type 2 diabetes in the general UK population is estimated using the Health Improvement Network database. Data are presented on treatment patterns in incident cases, and on body mass index in prevalent and incident cases.

2

The burden and risks of diabetic complications

Diabetes is responsible for approximately 4% of deaths globally (World Health Organization, 2010). In terms of morbidity, the World Health Organization (2010) reports that people with diabetes have a twofold increase in the risk of stroke (Boden-Albala et al., 2008), that diabetes is the leading cause of renal failure, that half of all nontraumatic lower limb amputations are due to diabetes (Icks et al., 2009), that diabetes is one of the leading causes of visual impairment and blindness in developed countries (Resnikoff et al., 2004), that people with diabetes require at least two to three times the health care resources compared to people who do not have the disease, that diabetes care may account for up to 15% of national health care budgets (Zhang et al., 2010) and that the risk of tuberculosis is three times higher among people with diabetes (Jeon and Murray, 2008).

It is clear that there are significant mortality and morbidity risks and burdens associated with diabetes; these

have been subdivided in this chapter into acute metabolic complications of diabetes, microvascular complications of diabetes and macrovascular complications of diabetes. Other possible health consequences of diabetes are then discussed (Box 2.1).

Acute metabolic complications of diabetes

Hypoglycaemia

People with diabetes are at risk of developing hypoglycaemia. This is when the amount of glucose in the blood decreases to a level that is insufficient to support the body (around less than 4 mmol/L). The brain is thus deprived of glucose needed for energy. Symptoms of hypoglycaemia include hunger, sweating, dizziness, tiredness, blurred vision, shakiness, irritability, going pale, fast pulse and difficulty in concentrating; there may be eventual progression to confusion and irrational behaviour and ultimately loss of consciousness.

> **Box 2.1 What are common consequences of diabetes?**
>
> Over time, diabetes can cause macrovascular complications (damage to the heart and blood vessels) and microvascular complications (damage to the eyes, kidneys and nerves).
> - Diabetes increases the risk of heart disease and stroke. Around 50% of people with diabetes die of cardiovascular disease.
> - Diabetic retinopathy is a common cause of blindness and occurs as a result of long-term accumulated damage to the small blood vessels in the retina. After 15 years of diabetes, approximately 2% of people become blind and about 10% develop severe visual impairment.
> - Diabetes is among the leading causes of kidney failure. 10–20% of people with diabetes die of kidney failure.
> - Diabetic neuropathy is damage to the nerves as a result of diabetes and affects up to 50% of people with diabetes. Although many different problems can occur as a result of diabetic neuropathy, common symptoms are tingling, pain, numbness or weakness in the feet and hands.
> - Combined with reduced blood flow, neuropathy in the feet increases the chance of foot ulcers and eventual limb amputation.
> - The overall risk of people dying with diabetes is at least double the risk of their nondiabetic counterparts.
>
> *Source: World Health Organization (2015).*

Patients with hypoglycaemia need access to an immediate source of glucose. Hypoglycaemic episodes are classified as mild (the patient can self-treat), moderate (the patient requires help from another individual) or severe (the patient begins to lose consciousness). Episodes can occur in people with diabetes if too much insulin has been administered or in the presence of other glucose-lowering drugs (especially sulfonylureas).

It has been estimated that people with type 1 diabetes experience on average around 43 symptomatic episodes of hypoglycaemia every year and up to two episodes of severe hypoglycaemia. People with type 2 diabetes who are treated with insulin have around 16 episodes every year and about one severe episode every 5 years (Perlmuter et al., 2008). Hypoglycaemia may also be implicated as a rare cause of sudden death in people with type 1 and type 2 diabetes.

The risk of hypoglycaemia increases with increasing duration of insulin treatment and previous history of hypoglycaemia. Hypoglycaemic unawareness occurs when people no longer notice the automatic warning signs of hypoglycaemia because their bodies become used to frequent periods of hypoglycaemia.

Diabetic ketoacidosis

Diabetic ketoacidosis (DKA) and hyperosmolar hyperglycaemic state (HHS; see below) are acute, life-threatening metabolic complications of diabetes, with a mixed presentation occurring in around one-third of patients (Kitabchi et al., 2006).

DKA occurs in the absence, or almost complete absence, of insulin and is characterised by the presence of hyperglycaemia, acidosis and ketosis. Lack of insulin causes hyperglycaemia and also stimulates the breakdown of fat and muscle as a fuel source, resulting in acidic by-products known as ketones (ketoacidosis). Symptoms of DKA include frequent urination and thirst, fatigue and signs of dehydration. Other symptoms may include nausea and vomiting, abdominal pain, confusion, rapid and laboured breathing, fruity-smelling breath and unconsciousness/coma. Patients with DKA require urgent treatment with insulin and with electrolyte and fluid replacement.

DKA is more common in type 1 diabetes, and around 5–15% of cases of DKA occur as the presenting symptom for type 1 diabetes. Other common causes are inadequate adherence (or nonadherence) to insulin treatment (around 15% of cases) and infection (30%). Although DKA rarely occurs in type 2 diabetes, it is recognised that people with type 2 diabetes from certain ethnic minority groups are prone to DKA (Kitabchi et al., 2006).

The mortality rate from DKA is less than 5%, but this increases with age. It has been estimated that the annual incidence rate is around 5–8 episodes per 1000 people with diabetes and accounts for up to 10% of hospital admissions in this group (Kitabchi et al., 2001). In the UK, 9% of children and young people with diabetes experienced at least one episode of DKA in 2009/2010 (Diabetes UK, 2012a).

Hyperosmolar hyperglycaemic state

HHS occurs in type 2 diabetes and is characterised by hyperglycaemia, hyperosmolarity and dehydration. Although insulin levels are insufficient to regulate glucose levels in the blood (which can become as high as 40 mmol/L), there is sufficient insulin to prevent the breakdown of fat and muscle, so ketoacidosis is avoided. Symptoms of HHS include weakness, leg cramps and visual impairment. There may also be signs of dehydration and disorientation.

Around 40% of cases of HHS occur as the presenting symptom for type 2 diabetes. Infection is another common cause, as are medications that increase glucose levels in the blood.

The mortality rate from HHS is around 15%, increasing with age and comorbidity, although HHS accounts for fewer hospital admissions than DKA (Kitabchi et al., 2006). The incidence rate is also lower, at less than 1 case per 1000 patient-years.

Microvascular complications of diabetes

Diabetic eye disease

Diabetic eye disease encompasses diabetic retinopathy, macular oedema, cataract and glaucoma, with diabetes the leading cause of blindness among people of working age (Diabetes UK, 2012a).

Diabetic retinopathy is the most common diabetic eye disease and occurs as a result of changes in the structure and function of small blood vessels in the retina. There are four progressive stages: stages 1–3 (mild, moderate and severe nonproliferative retinopathy) and stage 4 (proliferative retinopathy). To begin with, small swellings occur in the small blood vessels of the retina (microaneurysms), leading to some blood vessels becoming blocked. As this becomes more prevalent, the blood supply to the retina is reduced, so it sends signals to the body to grow new blood vessels. In stage 4, growth of new blood vessels along the retina is triggered. These vessels are fragile and can leak, leading to vision loss and blindness. Macular oedema is also present in about half of all cases of proliferative diabetic retinopathy, although it can occur at any stage. Fluid leaks into the macula of the eye, causing swelling and blurred vision.

Epidemiological evidence regarding the incidence and prevalence of retinopathy is difficult to summarise, given wide variation in the populations studied, the inclusion criteria used and the retinopathy status assessed. Williams et al. (2004) present evidence from a systematic review of 359 international studies. In the UK specifically, for people with type 2 diabetes, progression from no retinopathy to retinopathy and to proliferative retinopathy is given as 60 per 1000 patient-years and 7 per 1000 patient-years, respectively. The rates are higher in type 1 diabetes.

The prevalence of retinopathy among people newly diagnosed with type 1 diabetes is estimated to be less than 3%, but between 6.7% and 30.2% among people newly diagnosed with type 2 diabetes. Prevalence increases with increasing duration of diabetes, and overall estimates for any retinopathy range from 33.6% to 36.7% in type 1 diabetes and from 21% to 52% in type 2 diabetes. However, after 20 years, prevalence of retinopathy may be 100% in type 1 diabetes and 60% in type 2 diabetes. The prevalence of proliferative retinopathy is less than 2% in type 1 and type 2 diabetes and is around 6% for clinically significant macular oedema. These figures equate to 750,000 people with diabetes in the UK who have some degree of diabetic retinopathy, 180,000 with maculopathy and 25,000 who are blind (Minassian and Reidy, 2009).

Hyperglycaemia is the most important risk factor for both the incidence and progression of diabetic retinopathy and macular oedema, with a reduction in hyperglycaemia associated with reduced risk at all levels of hyperglycaemia and no evidence of a threshold effect (Klein et al., 2011). Large trials in type 1 and type 2 diabetes confirm the benefits of intensive glycaemic control for reducing the incidence and progression of retinopathy. High blood pressure may also be a risk factor for retinopathy, although evidence from trials is less convincing.

Diabetes is also associated with increased risk of cataract. People with diabetes are two to five times more likely to develop cataracts than people without diabetes (Klein et al., 1995), and this risk may be even higher in younger patients. Likely risk factors in patients with diabetes include increasing age, presence of any retinopathy, poor glycaemic control and duration of diabetes (Janghorbani et al., 2000).

Evidence suggests that an increased risk of primary open-angle glaucoma (the most common type of glaucoma) for patients with diabetes is also likely, although it has been argued that this increased risk may simply be attributable to increased surveillance among people with diabetes. A meta-analysis of 12 observational studies suggested that diabetes conferred around a 1.5-fold increased risk of glaucoma (Bonovas et al., 2004). The Nurses' Health Study confirmed this increased risk in women with type 2 diabetes (Pasquale et al., 2006), as did a large cohort study of patients with diabetes enrolled in a managed care network in the United States

(Newman-Casey et al., 2011). Risk factors are likely to include age, duration of diabetes and poor glycaemic control.

Diabetic kidney disease

Chronic kidney disease (CKD) is defined as reduced kidney function or the presence of kidney damage for at least 3 months regardless of kidney function. Diabetes is the leading cause of CKD in developed countries and is caused by changes in small blood vessels, making the kidney leaky and inefficient.

Kidney function is assessed by measuring glomerular filtration rate (GFR), with reduced kidney function usually defined as GFR < 60 mL/min per $1.3\,m^2$. Kidney damage is indicated by elevated excretion of urinary albuminuria, measured by the albumin-to-creatinine ratio (ACR). Microalbuminuria is defined as an ACR of 30–299 mg/g and macroalbuminuria as ACR ≥ 300 mg/g. There are five progressive stages of kidney disease, culminating in end-stage renal disease (stage 5).

Diabetes is associated with a twofold increase in the risk of microalbuminuria. In type 1 diabetes, the peak age of onset of nephropathy is around 10–15 years after diagnosis, with up to 45% of people with type 1 diabetes likely to develop clinically evident disease during their lifetime. In type 2 diabetes, around 3% of people have nephropathy at diagnosis, and 25% have microalbuminuria after 10 years. This gives overall prevalence figures of microalbuminuria of 17–21% in type 1 diabetes and 9–46% in type 2 diabetes (Pavkov et al., 2011). For any diabetic kidney disease, the rate of progression to the next stage is 2–3% per year. Diabetes is thus the most common cause of end-stage renal disease in the UK (Diabetes UK, 2012), with kidney disease accounting for 21% of deaths in type 1 diabetes and 11% of deaths in type 2 diabetes (Morrish et al., 2001).

The main risk factors for the development and progression of diabetic kidney disease are hyperglycaemia, dyslipidaemia, high blood pressure, duration of diabetes, age at diagnosis and smoking (Gross et al., 2005). Hyperglycaemia is a particular risk factor for development and progression of microalbuminuria, but less important at more advanced stages of nephropathy.

Neuropathy and lower-extremity disease in diabetes

Neuropathy, or nerve damage, is a common long-term complication of diabetes, affecting up to half of all people with diabetes (Diabetes UK, 2012). Patients may experience sensory neuropathy (including pain, numbness, tingling in the hands and feet and sensitivity to touch), motor neuropathy (affecting nerves to the muscles and causing muscle weakness and pain) and autonomic neuropathy (affecting involuntary responses of the intestine, bladder and penis). Autonomic neuropathy is associated with erectile dysfunction in over half of men with

diabetes, with diabetes conferring over twice the risk (Selvin et al., 2007). Low levels of physical activity, obesity and poor glycaemic control are all thought to be associated with increased risk of erectile dysfunction in men with diabetes (Chitaley et al., 2009).

Both neuropathy and peripheral vascular disease (PVD; see next section) are risk factors for the development of foot ulceration and lower extremity disease in people with diabetes, with neuropathy implicated in 80% of new foot ulcers (Boulton and Bowling, 2011). The following statistics indicate the scale of the problem in diabetes (Singh et al., 2005). The lifetime risk of developing a foot ulcer for a patient with diabetes is between 15% and 25%. The annual incidence rate ranges from 1.0% to 4.1% and the prevalence from 4% to 10%. People with diabetes are between 10 and 30 times more likely to undergo limb amputation compared to the nondiabetic population, and foot ulcers precede around 85% of these amputations. The age-adjusted annual incidence of lower limb amputations ranges from 2.1 to 13.7 per 1000 people with diabetes.

Macrovascular complications of diabetes

Cardiovascular disease

Cardiovascular disease (including myocardial infarction (MI), stroke and disorders of the circulation) is the most common cause of death in people with diabetes. In a multinational study of 4713 people in 10 countries, cardiovascular disease accounted for 44% of mortality in type 1 diabetes and 52% in type 2 diabetes (Morrish et al., 2001). On average, people with diabetes have around twice the risk of developing cardiovascular disease compared to the nondiabetic population (Meigs, 2010), and the risk appears to be generally higher for women (The Emerging Risk Factors Collaboration, 2010).

> **! Thinking point**
>
> Why do you think that cardiovascular disease is the most common cause of death in people with diabetes?

In a meta-analysis involving nearly 700,000 people in 102 studies, the hazard ratio for death from coronary heart disease associated with any diabetes was 2.31, and for nonfatal MI it was 1.82 (The Emerging Risk Factors Collaboration, 2010). After adjustment for known risk factors, the adjusted hazard ratio for all coronary heart disease was 1.87. The hazard ratio for MI conferred by type 2 diabetes was found to be 2.13 in men and 2.95 in women in a large UK-based study, decreasing with increasing age (Mulnier et al., 2008). However, this was as high as 5 in some groups. The risk is also particularly high in type 1 diabetes, with hazard ratios of 3.6 and 7.7 reported for major

cardiovascular events for men and women, respectively (Soedamah-Muthu et al., 2006).

People with diabetes also have an approximately twofold increased risk of stroke, compared to the nondiabetic population. The hazard ratios for ischaemic and haemorrhagic stroke estimated from the preceding meta-analysis were 2.27 and 1.56, respectively, reducing to 2.24 for ischaemic stroke after adjusting for known risk factors. Again, hazard ratios were higher for women (The Emerging Risk Factors Collaboration, 2010). Hazard ratios specifically in type 1 diabetes are similar, with estimates of 2.08 for men and 2.32 for women reported from a UK-based study (Mulnier et al., 2006a).

Evidence suggests that people with type 2 diabetes are also around twice as likely to develop congestive heart failure compared to their nondiabetic counterparts, with high blood pressure, poor glycaemic control, obesity and coronary heart disease the main independent risk factors (Nichols et al., 2004).

These high risks result in high prevalence of cardiovascular disease in people with diabetes. Even among newly diagnosed people with diabetes, the prevalence of ischaemic heart disease may be as high as 24% (Spijkerman et al., 2004). The American Heart Association estimate that the lifetime risk for people with diabetes of dying with some form of heart disease or stroke is at least 65% (American Heart Association, 2012).

The standard risk factors for cardiovascular disease in the general population (high blood pressure, dyslipidaemia, obesity and smoking) are also risk factors for cardiovascular disease in people with diabetes. In addition, several nontraditional or 'novel' risk factors have been identified: specifically measures of thrombosis (levels of albumin, fibrinogen and von Willebrand factor, factor VIII activity) and measures of inflammation (leukocyte count; Bertoni and Goff, 2011). However, although evidence suggests that hyperglycaemia is an important diabetes-specific risk factor for cardiovascular disease, this evidence is less compelling than it is for

microvascular complications (Conget and Gimenez, 2009).

PVD, another long-term complication of diabetes, is characterised by narrowing of the arteries, usually in the legs. People with diabetes have a two- to fourfold increased risk of PVD, with age, duration of diabetes, smoking and presence of neuropathy all risk factors in this group. There are difficulties associated with estimating the true prevalence of PVD in the diabetic population, although this may be as high as 29% (American Diabetes Association, 2003b), and up to 10% of people with diabetes may already have PVD when they are diagnosed (Spijkerman et al., 2004; Box 2.2 and Fig. 2.1).

Box 2.2 The Emerging Risk Factors Collaboration

Although numerous epidemiological studies have been carried out on risk factors associated with cardiovascular disease in people with and without diabetes, often these individual studies are too small to derive reliable estimates of risk associated with less common risk factors and in different circumstances and populations. The Emerging Risk Factors Collaboration has been designed to utilise data from such individual prospective cohort studies in a large meta-analysis of over 1.1 million participants of 104 cohort studies in predominantly Caucasian populations. The specific objectives of the Collaboration are to investigate in detail the associations between lipid and inflammatory markers* and nonfatal myocardial infarction or coronary death in people without cardiovascular disease at baseline. The studies have also provided reliable estimates of the effects of diabetes on cardiovascular risk.

*Triglycerides, HDL-C, LDL-C (and non-HDL-C), apolipoproteins A-I and B, lipoprotein(a), C-reactive protein, albumin and leukocyte count.
Source: The Emerging Risk Factors Collaboration (2007).

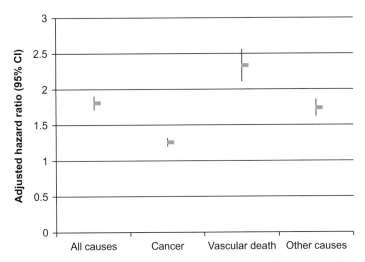

Fig. 2.1 *Hazard ratios, adjusted for age, sex, smoking and BMI, for different causes of death among people with diabetes derived from 820,900 people in 97 studies.*
Source: The Emerging Risk Factors Collaboration (2010).

Mortality from diabetes

On average, the risk of mortality is around twofold in people with type 2 diabetes compared to the general population (Mulnier et al., 2006b), and probably higher in type 1 diabetes (Asao et al., 2003; Wild, 2009). However, the relative risk varies by age and sex, ranging from 1.5 to around 6 depending on the demographic group. It decreases with increasing age and is generally higher in females (Roglic and Unwin, 2010). In contrast, the population attributable risk of mortality (the proportion of deaths in the population that would be avoided if diabetes were eliminated) increases with increasing age, as diabetes prevalence increases. Among adults aged 20–79 years, the overall proportion is estimated to 6.8% worldwide (Roglic and Unwin, 2010). In England more than 1 in 10 (11.6%) deaths among 20- to 79-year-olds can be attributed to diabetes. In some regions of the UK, approximately 1 in 8 (12.2%) of deaths among 20- to 79-year-olds could be attributable to the condition (YHPHA (2008)). Life expectancy is reduced, on average, by more than 20 years in people with type 1 diabetes and up to 10 years in people with type 2 diabetes (Diabetes UK, 2012a).

Deaths among people with diabetes occur as a result of acute metabolic

---

Box 2.3 Reporting of diabetes on death certificates

The use of death certificates to monitor deaths among people with diabetes and to thereby derive accurate mortality statistics among people with diabetes remains problematic. There are two parts to a death certificate. Part I shows the immediate cause of death and any underlying cause or causes. Part II shows any significant condition or disease that contributed to the death but that is not part of the sequence leading directly to death. However, if diabetes does not contribute to the cause of death, it is probably not appropriate to include diabetes on the death certificate.

Nevertheless, evidence shows that the proportion of death certificates with any mention of diabetes has remained consistently low over the past few decades, with analysis of temporal trends showing no improvement (Cheng et al., 2005; McEwen et al., 2011). In the United Kingdom Prospective Diabetes Study, 42% of death certificates of diabetic people mentioned diabetes (Thomason et al., 2005). In a study of the deaths of 1872 people with type 2 diabetes in Tayside, Scotland, even among people who died from cardiovascular disease, only 51% of their death certificates mentioned diabetes (Evans et al., 2008). Recording of type 2 diabetes on death certificates was particularly low among young people and those recently diagnosed. These figures have led to concerns that the underreporting of diabetes on the death certificates of diabetic people in different countries means that the true impact of diabetes on mortality is underestimated.

---

complications of diabetes or from longer-term complications. Patterns of mortality differ between type 1 and type 2 diabetes, with patients with type 1 diabetes more likely to die from renal disease, and those with type 2 diabetes from cardiovascular disease (Morrish et al., 2001).

Risk factors for increased mortality among people with diabetes include diabetes duration (after adjusting for age), low educational levels, ethnicity, smoking, treatment with insulin, high blood pressure, high cholesterol levels, hyperglycaemia and the presence of depression (Saydah and Eberhardt, 2011; Box 2.3).

! Thinking point

Diabetes UK argue that the number of deaths attributable to diabetes has consistently been underestimated. Why do you think this is?

Other consequences of diabetes

In addition to the established microvascular and macrovascular complications of diabetes, evidence suggests that a diagnosis of diabetes is also associated with a range of other adverse health consequences.

Diabetes and pregnancy

Diabetes in pregnancy can be classified into gestational diabetes (where the onset occurs during pregnancy) and preexisting type 1 or type 2 diabetes. Gestational diabetes accounts for the majority of diabetes in pregnancy (87.5%), with type 1 and type 2 diabetes accounting for 7.5% and 5%, respectively (National Institute for Clinical Excellence, 2008).

Diabetes in pregnancy is a growing public health concern. The incidence of gestational diabetes is increasing (Hunt and Schuller, 2007). Type 2 diabetes is also increasing in incidence and presenting in younger age groups (including women of childbearing age), thereby increasing the number of pregnancies complicated by preexisting diabetes. In the UK, 2–5% of pregnancies are complicated by diabetes. In California, between 1999 and 2005, 1.3% of pregnancies were complicated by preexisting diabetes and 7.6% by gestational diabetes (Lawrence et al., 2008). However, Reece et al. (2009) reported that the figure for gestational diabetes in the United States may be nearer 10%. Unplanned pregnancies are a particular concern, as it is important to have good glycaemic control even before conception to minimise the risk of developing diabetes-related complications during pregnancy.

Correa-Villasenor and Marcinkevage (2011) summarise the risks associated with diabetes in pregnancy. Women with preexisting diabetes at are increased risk of a range of adverse outcomes, including pregnancy-induced hypertension, preeclampsia, pyelonephritis and other infections, dyslipidaemia, preterm labour, caesarean delivery, acute metabolic complications of diabetes and worsening of longer-term complications. The offspring of mothers with preexisting diabetes are at risk of birth defects (including those of the cardiovascular, musculoskeletal and central nervous systems), intrauterine growth retardation, preterm birth, large for gestational age, birth trauma, asphyxia, respiratory distress syndrome, hypoglycaemia, stillbirth and perinatal mortality. Furthermore, the children of mothers with preexisting diabetes have increased risk of obesity and diabetes during adolescence. The frequency of these complications varies widely, but large for gestational age and preterm delivery may occur in at least one in four pregnancies of women with diabetes.

Although the risks of maternal and fetal complications associated with gestational diabetes are lower than those for preexisting diabetes, spontaneous preterm labour, induced labour and caesarean delivery are more common in women with gestational diabetes than in nondiabetic women. They are at increased risk of developing gestational diabetes in subsequent pregnancies and are at a sevenfold risk of developing type 2 diabetes (Bellamy et al., 2009). High proportions of women with gestational diabetes develop type 2 diabetes within 10 years (Kim et al., 2002). In terms of complications for their offspring, in addition to being large for gestational age, Reece et al. (2009) list infant respiratory distress syndrome, cardiomyopathy, hypoglycaemia, hypocalcaemia, hypomagnesaemia, polycythaemia and hyperviscosity. Furthermore, children of women with gestational diabetes are more likely to develop obesity, impaired glucose regulation and type 2 diabetes in later life.

Poorly managed diabetes is an important risk factor for many of these adverse outcomes in both preexisting diabetes and gestational diabetes, hence the need for good glycaemic control both before and during pregnancy (National Institute for Clinical Excellence, 2008). Unplanned pregnancy, delayed antenatal care and lack of or nonadherence to a diabetes management plan are therefore risk factors for these complications.

Diabetes and depression

Worldwide, 340 million people suffer from depression, including major depression, minor depression and dysthymia, and evidence from a wide range of studies indicates that the prevalence of depression is around twice as high in people with type 1 and type 2 diabetes compared to the nondiabetic population (Diabetes UK, 2012a). In the United States, Behavioral Risk Factor Surveillance Systems survey in 2006, the age-adjusted prevalence of depression among people with diabetes was estimated to be 8.3% (Li et al., 2008a). Worryingly, the prevalence of undiagnosed depression was thought to be similar.

The direction of causality between the coexistence of diabetes and depression is uncertain. It is possible that depression may be a risk factor for the development of diabetes, with the proposed causal mechanism being physiological changes arising from depression contributing to insulin resistance and beta cell dysfunction. Conversely, it has been suggested that the psychosocial stress of developing and living with diabetes causes depression. Egede and Ellis (2010) reported that depression is associated with a subsequent 60% increase in risk of type 2 diabetes, but that diabetes is associated with only a subsequent 15% increase in risk of depression.

However, regardless of the direction of causality, the coexistence of depression in people with diabetes is associated with poorer diabetes-related outcomes. Egede and Ellis (2010) noted that depression is associated with worse glycaemic control in both the short term and over longer periods of time, poor adherence to self-care regimens, the development of diabetic complications, disability, lowered work productivity and poorer quality of life. Effective treatment of depression in people with diabetes is therefore essential in diabetes management.

Diabetes in the older person

The prevalence of diabetes increases with age, with estimates of >10% in people over 65 years and >13% in people over 80 years (Wild et al., 2004), the majority of whom have type 2 diabetes. In a 12-year study of newly diagnosed type 2 diabetes in the Tayside region of Scotland, 45% of people were diagnosed when they were over the age of 65 (Barnett et al., 2010). A diagnosis of diabetes may be associated with a higher risk of age-related conditions among older people. These include physical disability, cognitive decline and dementia, urinary continence, depression, and falls and fractures (Volpato and Maraldi, 2011).

In a study of around 6500 adults over the age of 60 in the United States, Gregg et al. (2000) showed that diabetes was associated with a two- to threefold increased risk of being unable to do mobility-related tasks (walking for a quarter of a mile, climbing 10 steps, doing housework). Sinclair et al. (2008) noted a marked reduction in physical functioning among older people with diabetes in Wales. The biological mechanism for the association between diabetes and physical disability is likely to be multifactorial but all the following have been identified as possible risk factors: increased age and duration of diabetes, genetic predisposition, obesity, poor glycaemic control, peripheral arterial diseases, peripheral neuropathy, visual impairment, congestive heart failure, stroke, cognitive impairment, depression, arthritis, pain, poor

muscle quality and low-grade systemic inflammation (Volpato and Maraldi, 2011).

Diabetes is a risk factor for falls and fractures among older people, with over one-quarter of well-functioning older adults reporting falling each year in a study of health, ageing and body composition (Schwartz et al., 2008). Poor glycaemic control and the presence of diabetic complications (e.g. peripheral neuropathy, stroke, poor vision) are implicated in many falls. This can lead to an increased risk of fracture. Diabetes confers a 1.5- to 12-fold increased risk of hip fracture; fractures at other sites, including the humerus and spine, are also more common (Mayne et al., 2010).

Diabetes is associated with increased risk of urinary incontinence and lower urinary tract symptoms in women (Smith, 2006). Lower urinary tract symptoms (including urgency, frequency and nocturia) are also very common in men with diabetes.

Diabetes is a risk factor for cognitive decline and dementia. A review of 25 studies by Cukierman et al. (2005) suggested that the odds of cognitive decline were increased by between 1.2- and 1.7-fold for people with diabetes. There was a similar increased risk for dementia, with risks for both Alzheimer's disease and vascular dementia increased. The coexistence of diabetes and depression (discussed earlier) in older people is also very significant, given the high prevalence of both conditions in this age group (Boxes 2.4 and 2.5).

Box 2.4 The burden of diabetes and diabetic complications in Scotland

The Scottish Diabetes Survey annually collates data that are submitted by the 14 Health Boards in Scotland for all people with diabetes in a total population of around 5,200,000. This survey provides a picture of the national burden of diabetes and diabetic complications, and the following data were presented in the 2013 survey.

- There were 268,154 people in Scotland with diabetes: 5.0% of the total population. Of these people, 88% had type 2 diabetes, 11% had type 1 diabetes and 0.9% had other/unknown diabetes type.
- 37.5% of people with type 1 diabetes and 31.8% of those with type 2 diabetes (who had a BMI recorded) were overweight (BMI 25–30). The respective proportions for obesity (BMI > 30) were 24.8% and 55.0%.
- 88.7% of people with type 1 diabetes and 93.9% of those with type 2 diabetes had an HbA1c recorded. Of these, 21.5% and 61.1%, respectively, had HbA1c of < 58 mmol/mol (7.5%).
- 86.8% of those with type 1 and 94.9% of those with type 2 diabetes had their blood pressure recorded in the previous 15 months. Of these, 47.6% and 33.8%, respectively, had a systolic BP measurement of ≤130/80 mmHg.
- 3.6% of people with type 1 diabetes and 10.0% of those with type 2 diabetes had had a myocardial infarction and survived. 2.6% and 7.3%, respectively, had undergone cardiac revascularisation.
- 86.7% of people with diabetes had had eye screening in the previous 15 months.
- 1.2% of people with type 1 diabetes and 0.5% of people with type 2 diabetes had end-stage renal failure.
- 1.1% of people with type 1 diabetes and 0.7% of those with type 2 diabetes had had a lower limb amputation.

Source: Scottish Diabetes Survey Monitoring Group (2013).

Box 2.5 The burden of diabetes and diabetic complications in the United States

The figures presented here have been collated from several data sources by the Centers for Disease Control and Prevention (CDC), given that there is no national diabetes survey comparable to those carried out in some European countries. The data sources used include data systems of the CDC, the Indian Health Service's (IHS) National Patient Information Reporting System (NPIRS), the US Renal Data System of the National Institutes of Health (NIH), the US Census Bureau and other ad hoc studies. Numbers of people with diabetes were estimated from the 2005 to 2008 National Health and Nutrition Examination Survey (NHANES), the 2007–2009

Box 2.5 The burden of diabetes and diabetic complications in the United States–cont'd

National Health Interview Survey (NHIS), 2009 IHS data and US resident population estimates.

- 9.3% of the entire US population have diabetes.
- There were an estimated 28.9 million people over the age of 20 years with undiagnosed and diagnosed diabetes in 2012, representing 12.3% of the total population of this age.
- About 208,000 people younger than 20 years had diabetes. This represents 0.25% of all young people and includes type 1 and type 2 diabetes (of which the majority is type 1 diabetes).
- In 2011, 282,000 emergency room visits among adults over 18 years had a primary diagnosis of hypoglycaemia alongside a diagnosis of diabetes.
- In 2010, adjusted mortality rates for MI and stroke in adults with diabetes were 1.8 and 1.5 times higher respectively than among nondiabetic adults.
- In 2011, 228,924 people with diabetes and end-stage renal disease were on chronic dialysis or had had a kidney transplant.
- In 2005–2008, 4.2 million people with diabetes over the age of 40 years (28.5%) had diabetic retinopathy. 655,000 (4.4%) had advanced diabetic retinopathy.
- In 2010, about 73,000 nontraumatic lower-limb amputations were performed in people with diabetes.

Source: Centers for Disease Control and Prevention (2014).

 Summary points

- Hypoglycaemia is a common problem in people with diabetes.
- DKA and HHS are acute, life-threatening metabolic complications of diabetes. DKA is more common in type 1 diabetes, and each year around 9% of children and young people with diabetes experience an episode of DKA. HHS is more common in type 2 diabetes, but the incidence rate is lower.
- Diabetic eye is the leading cause of blindness among people of working age in the UK, with 750,000 people having some degree of diabetic retinopathy.
- Diabetes is the most common cause of end-stage renal disease in the UK. Kidney disease accounts for 21% of deaths in type 1 diabetes and 11% of deaths in type 2 diabetes.
- Neuropathy, or nerve damage, affects up to half of all people with diabetes.
- People with diabetes are between 10 and 30 times more likely to undergo limb amputation compared to the nondiabetic population.

Continued

Summary points—cont'd

- Cardiovascular disease is the most common cause of death in people with diabetes. On average, people with diabetes have around twice the risk of developing cardiovascular disease, compared to the nondiabetic population.
- The risk of mortality is around twofold in people with type 2 diabetes and higher in type 1 diabetes.
- Gestational diabetes and preexisting diabetes among pregnant women is a growing public health concern. Diabetes in pregnancy is associated with a range of complications for both the mother and the offspring.
- There is a high prevalence of depression in people with diabetes, and depression is associated with poor diabetes outcomes.
- In older people, diabetes is associated with an increased risk of physical disability, of falls and fractures, of lower urinary tract symptoms, and of cognitive decline and dementia.

Web pages and resources

http://www.cdc.gov/diabetes/statistics/complications_national.htm.
This Centers for Disease Prevention website presents comprehensive data on diabetes complications in the US.
http://www.who.int/chp/ncd_global_status_report/en/.
The WHO Global Status Report on Noncommunicable Diseases 2010 is the first report on the worldwide epidemic of diabetes and other NCDs, along with their risk factors and determinants. Chapter 1 is particularly useful.

Further reading

American Diabetes Association. Economic costs of diabetes in the US in 2007. Diabetes Care 2008;31:596–615.
This article presents the direct and indirect costs of diabetes and its complications in the United States in 2007. Although it is an American study, it provides a valuable insight into the huge economic burden incurred by diabetes.
The Emerging Risk Factors Collaboration. Diabetes mellitus, fasting glucose, and risk of cause-specific death. N Engl J Med 2011;364:829–41.
This article examines the extent to which diabetes mellitus or hyperglycaemia is related to risk of death from cancer or other nonvascular conditions. It is written as part of the Emerging Risk Factors Collaboration and is based on a study funded by the British Heart Foundation and others.

3 Management of diabetes and prevention of diabetic complications

Treatment of diabetes hinges on helping people with the condition to control their blood glucose levels and minimising their risk of developing complications over time. People with type 1 diabetes require treatment with insulin to control their glucose levels, whereas those with type 2 diabetes may be able to manage their condition through lifestyle management (diet and exercise) or by using oral blood glucose control therapies. However, some do require treatment with insulin. In this chapter, key points in the care and management of people with diabetes are discussed alongside individual-level interventions for the prevention of diabetic complications in people with diabetes.

Care and management of diabetes

The following key points in the care and management of children, young people and adults with type 1 diabetes are derived from the National Institute for Clinical Excellence (NICE) clinical guidelines 15 (National Institute for Clinical Excellence, 2004).

Care and management of diabetes in children and young people

Most people diagnosed with type 1 diabetes are under the age of 18 years. At diagnosis, children and young people should be offered a package of care from a multidisciplinary paediatric diabetes care team that includes expertise in clinical, educational, dietetic, lifestyle, mental health and foot care aspects of diabetes. They may be offered home-based or inpatient care depending on their particular circumstances. A structured programme of education should be offered at diagnosis that covers insulin therapy and delivery of insulin; self-monitoring of blood glucose; the effects of diet, physical activity and illness on glycaemic control; and the detection and management of hypoglycaemia. Provision of diabetes information and education should be an ongoing process.

There are three basic types of insulin regimen that are usually considered for young people. The most appropriate regimen will depend on the individual's age and circumstances. The insulin delivery system will also depend on insulin requirements and personal preference (e.g. short or long needles, depending on amount of body fat).

1. One, two or three insulin injections per day: These are injections mixed daily by the individual and are usually either short-acting (15 min to 2.5 h) or rapid-acting (30–60 min to 8 h) insulin analogues, mixed with intermediate insulin (1–2 to >16 h).

2. Multiple daily injections: These comprise injections of short-acting insulin or rapid-acting insulin analogue before meals, together with separate daily injection(s) of intermediate-acting insulin or long-acting insulin analogue (steady-state level after 2–4 days). Most young people are initially offered a multiple daily injection regimen. However, education, dietary management, instruction on the use of insulin delivery systems and self-monitoring, emotional and behavioural support, and clinical expertise in paediatric diabetes should all be part of the package of care that is delivered to a young person who is following such a regimen.

3. Continuous subcutaneous insulin infusion (CSII; insulin pump therapy): A young person may be offered insulin pump therapy if a multiple regimen has failed.

However, they need to have the commitment and competence to use it correctly.

The aim of insulin therapy (see Box 3.1) is to achieve a glycosylated haemoglobin (HbA1c) level (see Box 3.2) of <7.5% (58 mmol/mol), without frequent hypoglycaemia and to maintain a good quality of life. HbA1c should be tested two to four times per year, and young people must understand that low levels of HbA1c are associated

---

Box 3.1 Insulin pump therapy

An insulin pump, or continuous subcutaneous insulin infusion (CSII), is a programmable pump and insulin storage reservoir. It can provide a regular or continuous amount of insulin (usually rapid or short-acting) by a subcutaneous needle or cannula. Pumps can deliver varying amounts of insulin at a rate that is set by patients themselves and can also deliver additional doses when required. The pumps are small devices that are usually worn 24 h per day (although they can be removed for sports). They have a small plastic tube with a small needle or cannula at the end, which is inserted just under the skin and usually left for 2–3 days. Because patients programme the pumps themselves, according to diet, physical activity levels and results of blood glucose testing, this insulin delivery method does require competence, commitment and motivation from them.

Box 3.2 What is HbA1c?

The HbA1c test measures the amount of haemoglobin in the blood that is bound to glucose (glycosylated haemoglobin). People with persistently high blood glucose levels will have higher levels of HbA1c than people with normal blood glucose levels. Haemoglobin is carried by red blood cells, which have a lifespan of around 8–12 weeks. Therefore the HbA1c test is an indicator of the level of blood glucose control that has been achieved by an individual with diabetes over the previous 8–12 weeks.

HbA1c can be measured as a percentage (%) or in mmol/mol. The International Federation of Clinical Chemistry proposed a new reference method (mmol/mol) that is standardised across different countries. This was implemented in 2009. In the UK, HbA1c results are often still given by laboratories in both units.

In nondiabetic people, the HbA1c level is usually less than 6% (42 mmol/mol) of total haemoglobin. NICE clinical guidelines recommend the target HbA1c in people with type 1 diabetes to be <7.5% (58 mmol/mol) and in people with type 2 diabetes <6.5% (48 mmol/mol), without frequent episodes of hypoglycaemia.

Equivalent values for the old and new reference methods are as follows:

- 6.0% (42 mmol/mol)
- 6.5% (48 mmol/mol)
- 7.0% (53 mmol/mol)
- 7.5% (58 mmol/mol)
- 8.0% (64 mmol/mol)
- 9.0% (75 mmol/mol)

with increased risk of hypoglycaemia and that high levels are associated with increased risk of microvascular complications. Self-monitoring of blood glucose is recommended in people with type 1 diabetes (with preprandial targets of 4–8 mmol/L and postprandial targets of <10 mmol/L), who may be encouraged to adjust their insulin in response to readings.

The nutritional requirements and the importance of a healthy diet for a young person with type 1 diabetes are similar to those of a nondiabetic person, but they are likely to require dietetic support. Similarly, exercise is very important for the prevention of macrovascular complications; however, young people with type 1 diabetes need to be able to recognise and prevent exercise-induced hypoglycaemia. Self-monitoring may be recommended to help them understand the effects of exercise on blood glucose control.

In the case of hypoglycaemia, all people with type 1 diabetes must also have access to a source of carbohydrate (sucrose or glucose) for treatment, but severe hypoglycaemia usually requires hospital admission, as does the other major metabolic complication of diabetes, diabetic ketoacidosis. Children and young people with type 1 diabetes are also more likely to have emotional, behavioural and conduct problems, anxiety and depression, eating disorders (especially females) and cognitive disorders (especially if hypoglycaemic episodes occur frequently).

Adolescence is often a period of worsening glycaemic control. There should be specified local protocols for transferring young people from paediatric to adult care.

 Thinking point

Why might adolescence be a period of worsening glycaemic control?

Care and management of type 1 diabetes in adults

The management and care of adults who are diagnosed with type 1 diabetes is broadly similar to that for younger people. Adults require care from a multidisciplinary team, with an individual care plan that covers diabetes education (including nutritional advice), insulin therapy, self-monitoring, cardiovascular risk factor surveillance and management, surveillance and management of later diabetic complications, communication and follow-up/review. Adults should be offered a culturally appropriate structured programme of diabetes education, with a more formal review of their self-care and needs made annually.

For adults with type 1 diabetes, multiple insulin injection regimens may be offered as part of a package of care that includes education on nutrition and self-monitoring. These regimens again vary depending on the individual's needs and circumstances (e.g. whether isophane (NPH) insulin or insulin glargine is used). A twice-daily injection regimen, usually involving biphasic insulin preparations, is available for adults who are concerned about injection frequency. As with young people, adults may also be offered CSII (insulin pump therapy) if a multiple regimen has failed, and if they are sufficiently committed and competent. There may be particular circumstances, cultural or personal needs to be taken into account when selecting an insulin regimen: for example, whether the adult has learning difficulties and needs help to inject, whether they have nutritional and physical activity patterns that vary widely from day to day, or whether they have unusual patterns of eating, fasting and sleeping for religious or employment reasons. Similarly, the injection delivery system, including needle type, needs to be appropriate to the individual.

Adults with type 1 diabetes must understand that hypoglycaemia may sometimes be an unavoidable result of treatment with insulin. The choice of insulin regimen may therefore depend on the balance between avoiding hypoglycaemia but maintaining optimal blood glucose control.

The aim is for HbA1c to be less than or as near to 7.5% (58 mmol/mol) as possible. People with type 1 diabetes must understand that higher HbA1c is associated with increased risk of microvascular complications. HbA1c should be tested at least every 6 months. However, the benefits of HbA1c lower than 7.5% (58 mmol/mol) should also be made clear, particularly to people with a high risk of cardiovascular complications. Self-monitoring of blood glucose is recommended for adults with type 1 diabetes, with preprandial blood glucose level targets of 4.0–7.0 mmol/L and postprandial targets of < 9 mmol/L.

Adults with type 1 diabetes should be offered nutritional advice, both individually and as part of a structured diabetes education programme. They need to understand the effects of different foods on blood glucose levels so that they can make appropriate food choices and also understand how they might make changes to insulin doses in response. They need to be aware of the effects of alcohol, high-sugar and high-calorie foods, and foods with a high glycaemic index. Other important topics of education identified in NICE guideline 15 include glycaemic index of specific foods, body weight, energy balance and obesity management, cultural and religious diets, feasts and fasts, 'diabetic' foods, sweeteners, dietary fibre intake, protein intake, vitamin and mineral supplements, alcohol, matching carbohydrate, insulin and physical activity, salt intake in hypertension, comorbidities including nephropathy and renal failure, coeliac disease, cystic fibrosis or eating disorders, and the use of peer support groups.

As with young people, the benefits of exercise for the prevention of cardiovascular complications should be made clear to adults with type

1 diabetes. They may also need information on the appropriate intensity and frequency of physical exercise, the effects of exercise on insulin and nutritional requirements, how to adjust insulin doses in response to exercise and the role of self-monitoring in this.

Care and management of type 2 diabetes in adults

The following key points in the care and management of adults with type 2 diabetes are derived from the NICE clinical guideline 87 (National Institute for Clinical Excellence, 2009).

When a diagnosis of type 2 diabetes is made, it is essential that a structured education programme is offered, with annual reinforcement and review. This is particularly important given the lifestyle changes that are likely to be required, the central importance of self-care in managing type 2 diabetes and the general complexity of managing the condition. The education should be theory driven, evidence based and delivered by trained educators.

Initial management of type 2 diabetes is usually lifestyle or nonpharmacological management. Individuals require nutritional advice from a health care professional that is appropriate to their particular background and circumstances and also sensitive to their willingness to change. A healthy balanced diet for someone with type 2 diabetes is similar to that of a nondiabetic person: they require sources of carbohydrate that are high in fibre with a low glycaemic index (such as fruit, vegetables, whole grains and pulses). Low-fat dairy products and oily fish are encouraged, and the intake of foods containing saturated fat should be reduced. Dietary advice should be integrated with other aspects of lifestyle advice relating to increasing physical activity and losing weight, with an initial target for weight loss of 5–10% for people who are overweight. The target for HbA1c in people with type 2 diabetes is 6.5% (48 mmol/mol), and this should initially be measured every 2–6 months until it is stabilised, when 6-month checks are generally sufficient.

The next line of therapy for people for whom dietary and exercise lifestyle interventions do not result in adequate blood glucose control is oral blood glucose control therapies. Metformin is the recommended first-line treatment for people who are overweight. Sulfonylureas are usually considered for people who are not overweight or who do not tolerate metformin. A sulfonylurea may be added to metformin if blood glucose levels are not sufficiently controlled with metformin alone. Acarbose may also be used in people who cannot use other glucose-lowering medications. Other blood glucose control therapies that may be added in particular in circumstances when blood glucose levels are still not controlled include thiazolidinediones (pioglitazone and rosiglitazone), DPP-4 inhibitors (sitagliptin or vitagliptin), or GLP-1-mimetics (exenatide). Algorithms to guide choice of oral blood glucose therapy are provided in NICE and SIGN guidelines (National Institute for Clinical Excellence, 2004; Scottish Intercollegiate Guidelines Network, 2010).

When these medications still do not result in adequate blood glucose control, the individual may progress to insulin therapy. This may be in combination with oral agents, and again there is a range of possible insulin types and regimens. As in type 1 diabetes, it is very important that the regimen and insulin delivery system are appropriate to the individual and their particular lifestyle, with consideration given to factors such as whether assistance is required, whether hypoglycaemia is a problem, recreational activities and employment.

It is also essential that an individual receives further structured education when they commence treatment with insulin. This should include information on self-monitoring of blood glucose. Self-monitoring is not routinely recommended to people newly diagnosed with type 2 diabetes who do not use insulin because evidence for its effectiveness is not convincing. However, its use may be warranted in non-insulin-treated adults to provide information on hypoglycaemia to ensure safety during particular activities, when lifestyle or medication changes are made, or during illness.

Management of type 2 diabetes also involves considerable attention to the management of risk factors for microvascular and macrovascular complications (see following sections and Chapter 5).

Care and management of diabetes in pregnancy

The following key points in the care and management of diabetes in pregnancy are derived from the NICE clinical guideline 63 (National Institute for Clinical Excellence, 2008).

Diabetes in pregnancy is an increasing problem, with 2.5% of births in the UK involving women with diabetes. The majority of these births are complicated by gestational diabetes, but 7.5% involve women with preexisting type 1 diabetes and 5% with preexisting type 2 diabetes. The complications of diabetic pregnancy for mothers and their offspring are detailed in Chapter 2.

Preconception care in preexisting diabetes

Given the importance of good glycaemic control both before and during pregnancy for reducing the risk of diabetes-associated complications, unplanned pregnancy should be avoided in women with preexisting diabetes. Therefore this should be part of their diabetes education from adolescence. If they are planning a pregnancy, they should be offered a structured education programme and informed of the risks associated with diabetic pregnancy and the importance of good glycaemic control in reducing these risks. They also need to be aware of the risk of hypoglycaemia and hypoglycaemic unawareness during pregnancy, how nausea and vomiting may affect glycaemic control, and the need for assessment of retinopathy and nephropathy. They should be offered dietary advice, given advice on how to lose weight (if their BMI $> 27 \, kg/m^2$) and advised to take 5 mg of folic acid daily (until 12 weeks).

In general, women with diabetes who are planning a pregnancy should aim to achieve an HbA1c level of <6.5% (<48 mmol/mol) and to use contraception until good glycaemic control has been established. They should therefore be offered HbA1c measurement every month during the preconception period. Women with HbA1c of >10% (>86 mmol/mol) should be advised to avoid pregnancy. Glycaemic targets, frequency of glucose monitoring and diabetes medications should all be reviewed before and during pregnancy. Women may wish to commence or intensify glucose self-monitoring. In general, oral hypoglycaemic agents are discontinued before pregnancy and replaced with insulin, although some women may be offered metformin before and during pregnancy. Women should also be offered retinal and renal assessment.

Gestational diabetes

Risk factors for gestational diabetes (see Chapter 2) should be assessed in all pregnant women at the booking appointment, and they should be offered testing for gestational diabetes with an oral glucose tolerance test if there is at least one risk factor present (including a previous pregnancy complicated by gestational diabetes). When gestational diabetes is diagnosed, women should be offered information on the associated risks and the importance of good glycaemic control in reducing these risks. They also need to understand the role of diet, weight and exercise in reducing risk and given appropriate advice accordingly. Most cases of gestational diabetes do respond to changes in diet and exercise, although up to 20% of women may require treatment with oral hypoglycaemic agents or insulin. Such treatment should be considered if glucose targets are not achieved over a 1- to 2-week period or if there is evidence of macrosomia at diagnosis.

Antenatal, intrapartum and postnatal care

In general, pregnant women with diabetes should aim for fasting blood glucose levels of <5.3 mmol/L with postprandial targets 1 hour and 2 hours after meals of <7.8 mmol/L and <6.4 mmol/L respectively. Although individualised targets may be agreed. Women should monitor fasting blood glucose levels and postprandial levels 1 h after every meal, and those treated with insulin should also test before going to bed. The risks of hypoglycaemia and

hypoglycaemia unawareness should be understood by insulin-treated women in particular, who should also be provided with a concentrated glucose solution (and also glucagon in type 1 diabetes).

Women with diabetes should have regular contact with the diabetes care team throughout pregnancy (every 1–2 weeks) and offered continuing information and education. Antenatal examination of the fetal heart is offered at 18–20 weeks to screen for congenital malformations, with ultrasound monitoring every 4 weeks from 28 weeks. Women should be offered elective birth (induction of labour or elective caesarean section) after 38 weeks, and during labour and birth, capillary blood glucose should be maintained between 4 and 7 mmol/L. They should also be advised to give birth in a hospital where neonatal resuscitation is available.

After birth, if there is any indication of diabetes-associated complications, the baby should be admitted to the neonatal unit. Babies should have their blood glucose levels checked 2–4 h after delivery. The maternity unit needs to be alert to the risk of hypoglycaemia in the babies of women with diabetes. If blood glucose levels are <2 mmol/L on two separate occasions, the baby should be treated appropriately for hypoglycaemia. Women with diabetes also need to be aware of the effects of breastfeeding on their glycaemic control.

After delivery, women with preexisting diabetes can be referred back to routine diabetes care. Women with gestational diabetes need to be aware of the risk of gestational diabetes in any subsequent pregnancies, and of their future risk of type 2 diabetes.

Prevention of diabetic complications

As discussed in Chapter 2, common diabetic complications include the acute metabolic complications of diabetes and the microvascular and macrovascular complications of diabetes.

Prevention of acute metabolic consequences of diabetes

The key to prevention of acute metabolic consequences of diabetes is education and awareness raising. With regard to hypoglycaemia, patients need to be able to recognise early signs and symptoms and treat them appropriately. Conventional risk factors for hypoglycaemia are based on the assumption that hypoglycaemia is the result of insulin excess and include excess or wrongly timed insulin delivery, decreased insulin clearance (eg, due to renal failure), unusually low levels of glucose intake or decreased glucose production (eg, after alcohol intake), unusually high levels of glucose uptake (eg, during or after exercise) and increased insulin sensitivity (eg, at night). Patients therefore need some understanding of the physiologic processes underlying hypoglycaemia. An example of a structured education programme for patients with type 1

diabetes that has been shown to result in a reduction in severe hypoglycaemia and improved hypoglycaemic awareness is the DAFNE programme (Dose Adjustment for Normal Eating; Hopkins et al., 2012). A similar reduction in severe hypoglycaemic episodes was observed after evaluation of a structured group education programme among 1369 patients treated with insulin, including some with type 2 diabetes (Koev et al., 2003).

Prevention of diabetic ketoacidosis (DKA) and hyperosmolar hyperglycaemic state (HSS) may also be achieved by increasing awareness among patients and professionals of the early signs and symptoms of these conditions and an understanding of possible precipitating factors, such as infection or comorbidity. Kitabchi et al. (2006) also suggest that education around the signs and symptoms of uncontrolled diabetes, for primary care providers and those working with young people, might have the potential to reduce the incidence of DKA among cases of new-onset diabetes.

Prevention of microvascular complications

Strategies to prevent microvascular complications in type 1 and type 2 diabetes have generally focused on improving glycaemic control, as reflected in guidelines with fairly ambitious glycosylated haemoglobin targets. The Diabetes Control and Complications Trial (DCCT; see Boxes 3.3 and 3.4 for the UKPDS

Box 3.3 The Diabetes Control and Complications Trial: Prevention of microvascular complications

The Diabetes Control and Complications Trial (DCTT) was a large, multicentre randomized clinical trial conducted in 29 centres in the United States and Canada and funded by the National Institute of Diabetes and Digestive and Kidney Diseases. The trial was designed to compare the effects of intensive versus conventional diabetes therapy on the development and progression of complications in type 1 diabetes.

A total of 1441 patients aged 13–39 years, with type 1 diabetes (at that time referred to as IDDM: insulin-dependent diabetes mellitus), were recruited to the study between 1983 and 1989. Of these, 726 had diabetes duration of 1–5 years, had no evidence of retinopathy and had urinary albumin excretion < 40/24 h (the primary prevention cohort). The other 715 had diabetes duration of 1–15 years, evidence of mild to moderate nonproliferative retinopathy and had urinary albumin excretion of < 200 mg/24 h (the secondary prevention cohort).

Patients were randomised to either conventional therapy or intensive therapy. Patients in the conventional therapy cohort received one or two daily injections of insulin (but not daily adjustment of insulin dosage), daily self-monitoring of blood or urine glucose, and education on diet and exercise. They were examined every 3 months. Patients in the intensive therapy cohort received insulin three or more times daily by injection or external pump. The insulin dosage was adjusted according to dietary intake, anticipated exercise, and the results of self-monitoring of blood glucose that was carried out at least four times daily. These patients were examined monthly.

HbA1c and capillary glucose measures were statistically significantly lower in the intensive therapy cohort than in the conventional therapy cohort during the entire follow-up period. Forty-four percent of patients in the intensive therapy cohort achieved the target HbA1c of 6.05% or less at least once during the study (although the proportion whose mean value was less than 6.05% was very low (fewer than 5%)).

Over a mean follow-up of 6.5 years, the overall risk reductions (with 95% confidence intervals) that were observed were as follows:

- Development of *retinopathy* in primary prevention cohort: 70% (62–85%).
- Progression of *retinopathy* in secondary prevention cohort: 54% (39–66%).
- Development of *microalbuminuria* in primary prevention cohort: 34% (2–56%).
- Development of *microalbuminuria* in primary prevention cohort: 43% (21–58%).
- Development of *macroalbuminuria* in secondary prevention cohort: 54% (19–74%).
- Development of *neuropathy* in primary prevention cohort at 5 years: 69% (24–87%).
- Development of *neuropathy* in secondary prevention cohort at 5 years: 57% (29–73%).

The authors concluded that intensive therapy delays the onset and slows the progression of diabetic retinopathy, nephropathy and neuropathy in patients with type 1 diabetes. The DCCT provided a justification for pursuing tighter glycaemic control among patients with type 1 diabetes to reduce the risk of microvascular complications. However, there was an increased risk of hypoglycaemia in the intensively treated group.

Source: Diabetes Control and Complications Trial Research Group (1993).

Box 3.4 The United Kingdom Prospective Diabetes Study

The United Kingdom Prospective Diabetes Study (UKPDS) was a randomised controlled trial carried out in 23 hospitals in the UK between 1977 and 1991. Its aim was to determine the effects of intensive blood-glucose control (with either sulfonylurea or insulin) and conventional treatment on the risk of microvascular and macrovascular complications in patients with type 2 diabetes.

A group of 5102 patients between 25 and 61 years of age who were newly diagnosed with type 2 diabetes were recruited. Of 4209 eligible patients, nonoverweight patients were randomly assigned intensive treatment with insulin, intensive treatment with sulfonylurea or conventional treatment with diet (30%). Overweight patients were also randomly assigned these treatments, with a further alternative treatment of metformin. The goal of conventional treatment was to keep fasting plasma glucose < 15 mmol/L without symptoms of hyperglycaemia. The aim of intensive treatment was to keep fasting plasma glucose < 6 mmol/L and, in patients treated with insulin, preprandial glucose concentrations of 4–7 mmol/L.

In total, 1156 patients were intensively treated with insulin, 1579 patients were intensively treated with sulfonylureas, 1138 patients received conventional treatment and 342 overweight patients were treated with metformin. After around 10 years of follow-up, median HbA1c in the intensively treated group was 7.0%, compared with 7.9% in the conventional group. There was a statistically significant reduction in risk of microvascular complications of 25% in the intensively treated group. There was also a 16% reduction in risk of myocardial infarction (this included fatal and nonfatal myocardial infarction), but this result was not statistically significant.

Both the randomisation and the analyses in the UKPDS were relatively complex, but the study provided early evidence for the benefits of tight glycaemic control for the prevention of microvascular complications in type 2 diabetes.

Source: United Kingdom Prospective Diabetes Study Group (1998a).

---

trial) showed that lowering blood glucose with an intensive treatment regimen in type 1 diabetes reduced the risk of microvascular complications, including the development and progression of retinopathy, nephropathy and neuropathy (DCCT Research Group, 1993). The United Kingdom Prospective Diabetes Study demonstrated the benefits of improved glycaemic control in significantly reducing microvascular complications (particularly retinopathy) in patients with type 2 diabetes (American Diabetes Association, 2002). However, there is often a trade-off between tight glycaemic control and an increased risk of severe hypoglycaemia. Other strategies for prevention of specific complications are discussed in the following sections.

Diabetic eye disease

Although improving glycaemic control is key to preventing or delaying retinopathy, lowering blood pressure is also important. Otherwise, prevention of sight-threatening retinopathy in both type 1 and type 2 diabetes relies upon early detection of asymptomatic disease through screening. The aim of a screening programme is to detect disease before the usual time of diagnosis in individuals who do not yet have signs and symptoms of the disease to discover those among the apparently well who are in fact suffering from disease (Wilson and Jungner, 1968; see Chapter 6). Systematic screening in patients with diabetes involves digital photography of the retina followed by a two- or three-stage image grading process to identify the changes of sight-threatening diabetic retinopathy. This has around 80% sensitivity and 90% specificity for detecting sight-threatening lesions. In the UK, screening is offered at the time of diagnosis and then annually to people age 12 or over with diabetes.

However, screening uptake remains a considerable public health problem. In 2010/2011, 79% of 2,260,000 people in England who were offered screening for diabetic retinopathy took up the offer (NHS Diabetic Eye Screening Programme, 2012). In Scotland, the equivalent figure for the 2011/2012 period for 227,380 eligible people with diabetes was 76.7% (National Diabetes Retinopathy Screening, 2012). Perhaps more worryingly, Leese et al. (2008) showed that among over 16,000 people with diabetes in Tayside, Scotland, those who had the highest risks of retinal disease were those who were most likely to miss screening: younger age, poor glycaemic and blood pressure control, smoking, long duration of diabetes and social deprivation were all associated with low screening uptake.

> **! Thinking point**
>
> What might be done to encourage screening uptake for diabetic eye disease?

Diabetic kidney disease

Prevention of diabetic kidney disease in both type 1 and type 2 diabetes also relies on treatment of known risk factors. These include hyperglycaemia, although evidence for the benefits of tight glycaemic control is stronger for the incidence of microalbuminuria than for progression from microalbuminuria to macroalbuminuria and decline in renal function (Gross et al., 2005). Lowering blood pressure also has a significant effect on incidence and progression to microalbuminuria, for which a wide range of therapeutic agents is available.

Another strategy is the multifactorial approach, in which several risk factors are targeted simultaneously. In the STENO-2 trial, intensive treatment consisting of stepwise implementation of behaviour modification and pharmacological therapy targeting hyperglycaemia, hypertension, and dyslipidaemia was effective in slowing progression to nephropathy in patients with type 2 diabetes who had microalbuminuria, although not in those with type 1 diabetes (Gaede et al., 1999). Such multifactorial approaches are also likely to affect the incidence of cardiovascular complications.

The early detection of microalbuminuria in patients with diabetes is important to slow the progression of the disease. Annual screening for all patients with diabetes is therefore advised for estimation of the glomerular filtration rate and the albumin-to-creatinine ratio. Further investigation may then be required.

Neuropathy and lower-extremity disease in diabetes

Improving glycaemic control is important for reducing the incidence of neuropathy, as indicated by a recent systematic review (Callaghan et al., 2012).

Once a patient has diabetic neuropathy, appropriate foot care is crucial to prevent ulcers, infections and amputation. Education of patients and health care professionals is an essential part of this. Patients need to understand the implications of the loss of protective sensations in their feet; the importance of checking their feet daily for dry and cracking skin, calluses and signs of infection; and proper nail and skin care.

Suitable footwear that is correctly fitted is essential, and care should be taken with new shoes.

Clinical guidelines generally recommend annual foot examination for all patients with diabetes.

Prevention of macrovascular complications

The role of tight glycaemic control in the prevention of macrovascular complications is less convincing than that for microvascular complications. Although reductions in cardiovascular disease were associated with tight glycaemic control in patients with type 1 diabetes in the DCCT (DCCT/EDIC Research Group, 2005; see Box 3.5 and Box 3.6), the evidence from the United Kingdom Prospective Diabetes Study was less certain for type 2 diabetes (American Diabetes Association, 2002). The ACCORD trial among 10,251 middle-aged patients with type 2 diabetes was terminated early due to increased mortality in the intensively treated group and no evidence of a reduction in major cardiovascular events (ACCORD Study Group, 2008). More recently, the ADVANCE trial, carried out among over 10,000 people with type 2 diabetes in 20 countries, identified no significant reduction in cardiovascular disease (Heller et al., 2009). A meta-analysis of 13 trials in patients with type 2 diabetes found no benefit of intensive glycaemic control on mortality or death from cardiovascular causes (although a possible small reduction in nonfatal

---

Box 3.5 The Diabetes Control and Complications Trial and the United Kingdom Prospective Diabetes Study: Risks of hypoglycaemia

There was evidence of an increased risk of hypoglycaemia in the intensively treated cohort compared to the conventional cohort in the Diabetes Control and Complications Trial. For example, the incidence of severe hypoglycaemia was approximately three times higher. This result was statistically significant. There were 62 hypoglycaemic episodes per 100 patient-years where assistance was required in the intensively treated cohort, compared with 19 episodes per 100 patient-years in the conventional therapy group. This included 16 and 5 episodes of coma/seizure per 100 patient-years in each group respectively. Although there was no significant difference in the number of major accidents requiring hospitalisation (20 in the intensive therapy group and 22 in the conventional therapy group), there were two fatal road accidents, one in each group, in which hypoglycaemia might have been implicated. Forty patients receiving intensive treatment required a total of 54 admissions to treat severe hypoglycaemia, compared with 27 patients requiring 36 hospital admissions in the conventional therapy group.

Similarly, the United Kingdom Prospective Diabetes Study also drew attention to the risks of hypoglycaemia associated with intensive treatment. The proportions of patients with at least one major hypoglycaemic episode in a year, or at least any hypoglycaemic episode in a year, were significantly higher in the intensive group than in the conventional group. All hypoglycaemic episodes were most common in patients on insulin therapy.

These findings therefore emphasise the need to balance tight glycaemic control with minimising the risk of hypoglycaemia in intensively treated patients. However, there is evidence that high-quality skills training in insulin self-management can lead to improved glycaemic control without increasing severe hypoglycaemia.

Sources: Diabetes Control and Complications Trial Research Group (1993); United Kingdom Prospective Diabetes Study Group (1998a).

---

myocardial infarction was identified; Boussageon et al., 2012). Intensive treatment was associated with a twofold increase in severe hypoglycaemia. Given these findings, the focus has shifted toward multifactorial management of other cardiovascular risk factors, particularly those associated with the metabolic syndrome.

Lowering blood pressure in patients with type 2 diabetes is associated with reduced cardiovascular events and mortality. This was initially established by the United Kingdom Prospective Diabetes Study, where patients with tight blood pressure control had reduced risks of several diabetes-related endpoints, including

Box 3.6 The Diabetes Control and Complications Trial/Epidemiology of Diabetic Interventions and Complications Trial

In the DCCT/EDIC Trial, 93% of the original participants of the DCCT were followed up for a further 12 years to determine the effect of intensive treatment versus conventional treatment on the long-term incidence of cardiovascular disease. However, at the end of the DCCT, all patients were offered intensive treatment and they returned to their usual health care providers for their treatment. During the subsequent 11-year period, differences in treatment and in HbA1c diminished between the two groups. Overall, the intensive treatment cohort had mean HbA1c of 8.0%, compared to 8.2% in the conventional treatment cohort.

However, the risk reduction associated with even this 6.5-year period of intensive treatment was 42% (95% confidence interval 9–63%) for any cardiovascular disease and 57% (12–79%) for nonfatal myocardial infarction, stroke or death from cardiovascular disease.

Source: The Diabetes Control and Complications Trial/Epidemiology of Diabetes Interventions and Complications (DCCT/EDIC) Study Research Group (2005).

inhibitors, calcium channel blockers and angiotensin-II receptor antagonists all commonly used. Patients should have their blood pressure checked at least annually.

Improving lipid profile is another approach to reducing the risk of cardiovascular disease. Statins are used to reduce LDL cholesterol, and their subsequent significant effects on reducing the risk of cardiovascular events have been shown in trials such as the Heart Protection Study and the CARDS Trial (Adler, 2011). Fibrates raise HDL cholesterol levels and lower the concentration of triglycerides, although the evidence for reducing cardiovascular events is less strong. Nevertheless, fibrates are recommended if serum triglycerides are very high (National Institute for Clinical Excellence, 2009).

Low-dose (75 mg) daily aspirin (antithrombotic therapy) may be offered to patients at high risk of cardiovascular events, and several trials are currently underway to determine whether this significantly reduces their incidence (Adler, 2011).

Lifestyle modification, including dietary changes such as reducing intake of saturated fats and cholesterol and increasing dietary fibre, and reducing body weight, increasing physical activity and stopping smoking, remain key aspects of diabetes management. Although formal evidence for their effects on reducing the risks of specific diabetic complications may be patchy (Nield et al., 2007), effects on intermediate outcomes (eg, blood

a 44% reduction in stroke (UKPDS, 1998b). Multiple drug therapy may be required to reduce blood pressure, with angiotensin-converting enzyme (ACE) pressure) are well established. From a public health point of view, promotion of a healthy lifestyle is entirely justified.

Risk estimation tools

Risk estimation tools are used to stratify people according to their risk of a subsequent disease. This may then help clinicians to target people at highest absolute risk of an outcome, to select appropriate therapies, to provide prognostic information or to motivate patients to make behavioural changes. They are developed using multivariate equations, and risk is estimated according to the values/levels of specific risk factors. For example, the Framingham Risk Score Equation is probably the most well known. It is freely available on the Internet and can be used by any individual to determine their risk of having a heart attack in the next 10 years (see Web pages and resources).

Chamnan et al. (2009) identified 17 different risk scores for use in people with diabetes to predict their risks of cardiovascular disease, coronary heart disease and cerebrovascular disease or stroke. Some, such as the Framingham Risk Score Equation, were developed in the general population, and these generally include a binary variable as to whether or not a person has diabetes. Others have been developed in populations of people with diabetes and include diabetes-specific risk factors, such as glycaemic control or duration of diabetes.

Although the predictive performance of the risk scores varied widely between different populations, diabetes-specific risk scores did not appear to perform significantly better than those developed in general populations. However, in general, risk scores ranked individuals reasonably accurately, which is important in identifying high-risk patients. However, Chamnan et al. (2009) argue that unless absolute risk estimation (rather than relative risk estimation) is very accurate, care should be taken when using the results to communicate prognostic information to patients.

The use of the UKPDS risk engine is recommended for estimation of cardiovascular risk in the UK (National Institute for Clinical Excellence, 2009). A recent validation study suggested overestimation of the true risk among people with diabetes (Simmons et al., 2009).

✏️ Summary points

- The central aim of diabetes management is to help people control their blood glucose levels and to minimise the risk of diabetic complications over time.
- People with diabetes require care from a multidisciplinary team that has expertise in all aspects of diabetes, and a structured programme of education should be available to them when they are diagnosed.

Summary points—cont'd

- People with type 1 diabetes require treatment with insulin. The most appropriate insulin regimen will depend on the individual's particular circumstances and lifestyle.
- Lifestyle or nonpharmacological management may be appropriate for some people with type 2 diabetes. If this does not result in an adequate blood glucose control, the next line of therapy is treatment with oral blood glucose control agents. Many people with type 2 diabetes eventually progress to insulin therapy.
- Good glycaemic control is essential for women with preexisting diabetes or who develop gestational diabetes during pregnancy to minimise the risk of diabetes-associated complications. The importance of avoiding unplanned pregnancy needs to be made clear to women with preexisting diabetes from adolescence.
- Increasing awareness and education among people with diabetes, and also the general population, are needed to prevent acute metabolic complications of diabetes.
- Improving glycaemic control and lowering blood pressure are key strategies to prevent the development of retinopathy. The early detection of asymptomatic disease through screening is also important, although low and differential screening uptake remains a considerable problem.
- Improving glycaemic control and lowering blood pressure are important for reducing the incidence of diabetic kidney disease. The early detection of microalbuminuria by annually screening all people with diabetes is generally recommended.
- Improving glycaemic control is important to reduce the incidence of neuropathy. Once neuropathy is diagnosed, education of people in appropriate foot care is the main strategy for prevention of ulcers, infections and amputation. All people with diabetes should have annual foot examinations.
- The role of improved glycaemic control is less certain in the prevention of macrovascular complications. Multifactorial management of other cardiovascular risk factors, particularly those associated with the metabolic syndrome, is advocated for the prevention of macrovascular disease.
- Risk estimation scores are available to predict cardiovascular risk in people with diabetes to identify those that are at highest risk.

Web pages and resources

National Institute for Clinical Excellence. Clinical guideline 15. Type 1 diabetes: diagnosis and management of type 1 diabetes in children, young people and adults; 2004. http://guidance.nice.org.uk/CG15/NICEGuidance/pdf/English.

National Institute for Clinical Excellence. Clinical guideline 63. Diabetes in pregnancy. Management of diabetes and diabetic complications from pre-conception to the postnatal period; 2015. https://www.nice.org.uk/guidance/ng3.

National Institute for Clinical Excellence. Clinical guideline 87. Type 2 diabetes. The management of type 2 diabetes; 2012. http://www.nice.org.uk/CG87.

Scottish Intercollegiate Guidelines Network. 116. Management of diabetes. A national clinical guideline; 2010. http://www.sign.ac.uk/pdf/sign116.pdf.

These guidelines summarize best practice in the care of people with diabetes, alongside the level of the evidence supporting them.

Diabetes Trials Unit, University of Oxford. The UKPDS risk engine. http://www.dtu.ox.ac.uk/riskengine/.

National Cholesterol Education Program. Risk assessment tool for estimating your 10-year risk of having a heart attack. http://hp2010.nhlbihin.net/atpiii/calculator.asp.

Further reading

Chamnan P, Simmons RK, Sharp SJ, Griffin SJ, Wareham NJ. Cardiovascular risk assessment scores for people with diabetes: a systematic review. Diabetologia 2009;52:2001–14.

This review compares and contrasts 17 different cardiovascular risk scores used in people with diabetes.

Mahmud M, Mazza D. Preconception care of women with diabetes: a review of current guideline recommendations. BMC Womens Health 2010;10:5.

This paper provides an interesting discussion of the consistency of different international guidelines on the preconception care of women with diabetes.

Mazzola N. Review of current and emerging therapies in type 2 diabetes mellitus. Am J Manage Care 2012;18:S17–26.

This is an American review written by a pharmacist and provides information on the range of pharmaceutical agents used to treat diabetes, including updates on the newest drugs available.

Zimmet P. Preventing diabetic complications: a primary care perspective. Diabetes Res Clin Pract 2009;84:107–16.

This article provides some general information on the burden and treatment of diabetic complications; it also discusses findings arising from the Fenofibrate Intervention and Event Lowering in Diabetes (FIELD) Trial.

4 Organisation of diabetes care

Models of diabetes care

Given the complexity of the condition, a person with diabetes is likely to require access to a range of different services during their lifetime (see Box 4.1 for an example of some of these services). During the period immediately after diagnosis with type 2 diabetes, the individual needs to have the knowledge and skills to self-manage their condition effectively in partnership with health care professionals, hence the importance of structured education at this point. After this first year, continuing care needs to be established. This is the cycle of regular recall, review and renegotiation of care. As the disease progresses, it is likely that an individual with diabetes will need increasing access to more specialist services in response to events such as pregnancy, hospital admission, metabolic complications, development of longer-term complications and disability. Given the many components of an effective diabetes service, how this service is organised is an important question.

Fifty years ago, a person with diabetes would have been treated in hospital solely by one specialist. However, once the increasing prevalence of diabetes necessitated the involvement of primary and community health care professionals in diabetes care, the importance of collaboration between primary and secondary care was recognised and led to the development of the shared care model. Shared care is defined as 'the joint participation of primary care physicians and specialty care physicians in the planned delivery of care, informed by an adequate education programme and information exchange over and above routine referral notices'. A national survey of the organisation of diabetes care in England and Wales in 2000 indicated that at that time over half of a national sample of 1320 general practices (GPs) operated a formal shared care protocol with a local diabetes specialist team and met regularly with its members (Pierce et al., 2000).

Box 4.1   The key characteristics of an integrated diabetes service, as outlined in the report 'Commissioning diabetes without walls' (NHS Diabetes, 2009)

- Maximise opportunities for preventing complications of diabetes through an effective empowerment and partnership approach, focusing on individual care planning, support for professional and patient education, and emotional and psychological care.
- Provide appropriate specialist care when and where it is convenient to the person with diabetes (care closer to home).
- Provide early proactive intensive care of at-high-risk cases with early complications.
- Provide a multidisciplinary approach using effective communication across boundaries and specialties.
- Provide a service commissioned on use of competencies, not roles, to deliver care.
- Provide improved inpatient care, by responding to the requirements of the person with diabetes and to reduce their length of stay in hospital regardless of the reason for admission.
- Reduce amputations through improved awareness and treatment by ward staff.
- Provide a safe use of insulin/prescribing whatever the context.
- Provide early information and specialist diabetes support for preconception and pregnancy for women who have diabetes.
- Ensure children and young people and their families using services are informed and empowered to take control of their care.
- Ensure children and young people and their families using services experience a smooth transition into adult services through professionals working across boundaries to ensure this happens.
- Provide dignity and respect to older people with diabetes and offer a multidisciplinary service to meet individual needs.

Source: NHS Diabetes (2009).

The favoured model for diabetes care is now an integrated approach to the planning and delivery of care. Integrated care is an organising principle for care delivery with the aim of achieving improved patient care through better coordination of services provided (Shaw et al., 2011). As outlined in a Joint Position Statement (Diabetes UK et al., 2007), the integrated approach prioritises the needs of the individual, rather than the needs of the health care system, and aims to ensure that an individual's experience with different components of the health care system is 'seamless' and 'continuous'. The approach recognises the multiple interactions required between an individual with diabetes and primary, community, specialist and social care services and views a patient with diabetes as an active participant over a lifetime of care. There is also an emphasis on supporting self-care and meeting national standards of care. This means that health care professionals must work in partnership; they need to be aware of all the interactions that take place between a patient with diabetes and members of the health care team, and this needs to be supported by shared record keeping and technological solutions. The exact nature of an integrated care service may vary from location to location, but local models of integrated care should be informed by local standards and principles. Integrated care may be provided in different ways. Box 4.1 describes key characteristics of an integrated diabetes service for type 1 and type 2 diabetes. Corrigan et al. (2012) describe a model of integrated GP-led care in Bexley.

Managed clinical networks

One approach to the delivery of an integrated care service is a managed clinical network (MCN). An MCN is a linked group of health professionals and organisations from primary, secondary and tertiary care, working in a coordinated manner, unconstrained by existing professional and Health Board boundaries, to ensure equitable provision of high-quality clinically effective services. The integration is virtual rather than structural, in that it relies on clinicians being part of a virtual organisation that actively involves patients in service design. In Scotland, an MCN for diabetes care has been established in each of the 14 Health Boards, underpinned by the original key aims and principles as set out by the Scottish Executive Health Department (2002; see Box 4.2). An evaluation of a MCN set up in NHS Tayside suggested that it resulted in

---

Box 4.2   Key points from the core principles of an MCN as set out by the Scottish Executive Health Department (2002)

- MCNs must be managed with clear structures and lines of responsibility. A clinician or a clinical manager should take a lead role.
- The purpose of the networks is to improve patient care.
- Work undertaken must be evidence-based.
- Outcomes need to be measured.
- A quality assurance programme is required.
- Each network must produce a written annual report available to the public.
- Networks must be multidisciplinary and multiprofessional.
- Patients must be involved in shaping the network.
- MCNs should provide a mechanism for patients and clinicians to be involved in disease-specific planning and strategic thinking.

improvements in simple processes of care and in some intermediate outcomes, particularly in type 2 diabetes (Greene et al., 2009). The role of information technology was central to the success of the MCN.

Thinking point

Why would information technology be central to the success of the MCN?

Diabetes registries

Over the last two decades or so, UK government policy has increasingly supported the use of disease registries to improve care and to monitor and prevent ill health. A disease registry is a record of all instance of a disease within a defined area or a defined denominator population and is usually longitudinal in that information about individuals is updated regularly. From a public health point of view, a disease registry can be invaluable for epidemiological research (eg, for measuring the amount of disease in a population and examining trends over time, or for evaluating outcomes associated with different interventions), for clinical audit and for service organisation and evaluation. Registries can also have an important role in chronic disease management. Whereas paper-based registries have been used in the past, the development of computerised versions has greatly enhanced their potential and efficiency. For example, registries might be used to generate reports about clinical endpoints

in patients, to identify patients who are not receiving care according to specified protocols or guidelines, to create reminders of patient management tasks for both patients and clinicians, for facilitating call and recall and to create lists of patients who are at high risk of particular outcomes. A clinical database differs slightly from a disease registry in that it is usually a register of cases of a particular disease treated in one (or more) institution, and there is not necessarily a defined denominator population.

Given that diabetes is a lifelong disease, with multidisciplinary care that involves an array of care processes and standards, potential uses of a diabetes registry are manifold. It was advocated in the delivery strategy of the UK National Service Framework for Diabetes that all people diagnosed with diabetes should be identified in an up-to-date practice-based diabetes register (Department of Health, 2002). Although substantial progress has been made, there are still only a few countries in Europe that have comprehensive national diabetes registries, and these vary both in function and in quality and completeness (International Diabetes Federation, Europe, 2011) (see Boxes 4.3 and 4.4 for examples of National Disease Registries [NDRs]).

Thinking point

Why have so few countries developed a diabetes registry?

Box 4.3   Case study. National Diabetes Registry (NDR): two different approaches in Scandinavia

Denmark

Denmark has a population of 4,013,250 and a prevalence of diabetes of 8.6% in adults 20–79 years old. The NDR was established in 2006 by the National Board of Health. It is not based on direct reporting but uses existing national datasets to identify people with type 1 and type 2 diabetes. These datasets include the Danish Civil Registration System (DCRS), the National Patient Register (NPR), the National Health Service Register (NHSR) and the Danish National Prescription Register (DNPR; since 2007). The NDR is updated annually. An individual is entered on the NDR if:

- there is a diagnosis of diabetes on the NPR
- there is registration as a diabetic patient for chiropody on NHSR
- there are records of either two blood glucose measurements per year for five consecutive years or five blood glucose measurements in 1 year, on the NHSR, or
- there are records of purchase of insulin or oral antidiabetic medication (excluding metformin prescribed on its own to women 20–39 years old) on the DNPR.

It is estimated that the Danish DNR has coverage of 90%. There were 410,882 patients registered in 2008 (including patients who have died since being entered on the register). The register is thus a valuable resource for population-based studies in diabetes epidemiology.

Sweden

Sweden has a population of around 9 million and a prevalence of diabetes of 6.4% in adults 20–79 years old. The NDR was launched in 1996 and is maintained by the Swedish Society of Diabetology. It relies on the collection of clinical information relating to patients with type 1 and type 2 diabetes from clinical departments of medicine and primary health care centres. All clinical units are invited to participate, but this is not mandatory. The NDR has been online for data collection since 2002, and it is estimated that it covers around 50–60% of all patients with diabetes in Sweden. There were 346,679 patients entered on the NDR in 2012 (including patients who have died since being entered on the register), 296,122 being registered via primary care and 50,557 through hospitals. The main function of the Swedish NDR is to collate clinical data on patients with diabetes, and it is therefore more akin to a clinical database. It is thus particularly suited to studies on quality improvement and assessment of interventions within the diabetic population, rather than population-based epidemiology.

Box 4.4   Case study. The Scottish Care Information–Diabetes Collaboration

The Scottish Care Information–Diabetes Collaboration (SCI-DC) was launched on a national level in 2002 for the entire population of Scotland (over 5 million). This is a real-time web-based clinical information system for all patients with diabetes in Scotland that functions effectively as a disease register of all people with diabetes in Scotland and as a clinical database. The system captures data daily from over 1050 general practices (GPs) in Scotland and all 40 hospital clinics, covering all key clinical processes and events, including laboratory results and retinopathy screenings; there are also automatic updates of GP registration details and demographic information (such as date of death), ensuring that the diabetic population is accurately defined. The SCI-DC has multiple uses.

SCI-DC serves as a **shared electronic record** for individual patients that can be accessed by any health care professional involved in their care. Thus a clinician can view the details of all the care that their particular patient has received. For example, a hospital doctor can view records of drugs that have been prescribed in primary care. A GP can access information on any care provided in a hospital. This clearly supports multidisciplinary working and improved communication. SCI-DC also has **risk stratification** tools to enable clinicians to identify patients who may be at high risk of particular outcomes.

SCI-DC provides the facility to **audit** care at practice, regional and national levels to ensure that quality standards are met. It also serves as a portal for **dissemination of educational material** for patients and for care guidelines for health care professionals. Patients can also be trained to access parts of their own health records.

SCI-DC is an excellent platform to facilitate national **research** in diabetes. The Scottish Diabetes Research Network has been funded since 2006, with one of its key functions to carry out anonymised **epidemiological research** in diabetes using SCI-DC and other routine datasets. The SDRN Epidemiology Group has already published studies at the Scottish population level (Colhoun and the SDRN Epidemiology Group, 2009). As part of SCI-DC, a **national diabetes research register** has also been set up. This is a register of over 6000 consenting patients who have agreed that they can be contacted directly about research for which they are eligible. **GoDARTS** is another resource, initially funded by the Wellcome Trust and supported by Diabetes UK, that is recruiting around 10,000 consenting patients with type 2 diabetes and matched nondiabetic controls, who are then genotyped. This resource is helping to define genetic factors related to diabetes, including susceptibility, complications and response to treatment.

> **Box 4.4   Case study. The Scottish Care Information–Diabetes Collaboration—cont'd**
>
> **The DARTS diabetes register**
>
> SCI-DC had its early roots in a diabetes register that was developed in the 1990s for the region of Tayside, in Scotland, which has a population of around 400,000. This was known as the 'DARTS' diabetes register and used record-linkage techniques to gather data from various sources to identify people with diabetes (Morris et al., 1997). This was made possible through the widespread use of a unique 10-digit identifier, known as the CHI number, for all people registered with GPs in Tayside. The existence of an electronic dataset of all prescriptions dispensed to people in Tayside that had been developed for pharmacoepidemiological research also enhanced the sensitivity of the identification of people with diabetes. Although the regional DARTS diabetes registry has now been superseded by the national SCI-DC registry, the existence of historical data for the Tayside region dating back to the early 1990s has proved to be an excellent resource for longitudinal, epidemiological studies in type 1 and type 2 diabetes.

The diabetes care team and their roles

The GP is usually a patient's first point of contact with their health care team, with around three-quarters of patients with diabetes diagnosed in primary care. The majority of type 2 diabetes care in the UK is now led by primary care.

The role of a practice nurse is to deliver care and services within the GP or population setting. As such, many patients with diabetes receive diabetes-related care from their practice nurse, ranging from provision of advice, information and education to physical checkups.

Diabetes specialist nurses (DSNs) have specific expertise and training in the care of people with diabetes and work with this patient group only, assisting them to self-manage their diabetes effectively.

A survey in 2010 indicated that around one-half of DSNs work solely in hospital settings, with around two-thirds of inpatient settings having access to a DSN (Diabetes UK, 2014). Twenty percent were based in the community only. The majority of training courses for patients on diabetes self-management are delivered by DSNs. Paediatric DSNs provide similar care exclusively to children and young people with diabetes.

Consultant physicians/diabetologists have a special interest in diabetes and provide multidisciplinary diabetes specialist teams with leadership. The majority are based in acute hospitals, but some are employed to deliver and coordinate services in the community. Whether or how often a patient sees a diabetes consultant depends on how care is organised in their local area.

Diabetes specialist dieticians work as members of multidisciplinary teams across a variety of health care settings, including primary and secondary care. Their role is to provide specialist evidence-based dietary advice to patients with diabetes, taking into consideration other factors including nutritional status, medication, diabetes control and lifestyle.

Treatment and management of sight-threatening diabetic retinopathy is carried out by ophthalmologists. It is recommended that patients should undergo eye screening when they are diagnosed with diabetes and annually thereafter; this is mainly done by optometrists.

Current guidance recommends that diabetes specialist podiatrists are members of the health care team to undertake foot screening examinations and educate patients with diabetes and other health care professionals on the importance of foot health.

Other members of a diabetes care team might include psychologists, pharmacists and other medical specialists.

Quality of diabetes care

Quality of health care was defined by the Institute of Medicine in 2001 as 'the degree to which health services for individuals and populations increase the likelihood of desired health outcomes and are consistent with current professional knowledge'. Much of our current thinking on the assessment of quality in health care is underpinned by the work of Donabedian, who developed the framework of structure, process and outcome. In terms of diabetes, we can see how an effective structure (such as the existence of a diabetes registry) might influence effective processes (such as a patient identified on a registry having HbA1c measured regularly), which then has an impact on outcomes. Process measures are the most frequently used indicators of quality of care, partly because they are often easier to collect, although those that have been associated with clinical outcomes are obviously preferred. They also need to be simple to monitor and interpret.

The World Health Organization recognises six dimensions of quality in health care: that it is effective, efficient, accessible, acceptable/patient-centred, equitable and safe. In response to the increasing prevalence of diabetes and a recognition that diabetes care was suboptimal for many patients, attention in the 1990s began to be focused on developing suitable and reliable performance measures to assess the quality of diabetes care. The aim of the Diabetes Quality Improvement Project in the United States was to develop a set of measures that could be used across different health care systems and in different populations (Fleming et al., 2001). In the UK, the National Institute for Clinical Excellence has recently published quality standards for diabetes care for adults with diabetes that support the National Diabetes

Framework's standards (NICE, 2011a). They are achievable markers of high-quality cost-effective care, which are informed by evidence and based on three dimensions of quality: clinical effectiveness, patient safety and patient experience (see Box 4.5). However, there remain concerns that there is wide variation in standards of care, with many people with diabetes not receiving the standards of care that they should, and with significant regional variations. For example, only 49% of registered patients in the National Diabetes Audit received all nine of the recommended care processes at their annual review (National Audit Office, 2012).

Box 4.5   Quality standards set for adults with diabetes

- People with diabetes and/or their carers receive a structured educational programme that fulfils the nationally agreed-on criteria from the time of diagnosis, with annual review and access to ongoing education.
- People with diabetes receive personalised advice on nutrition and physical activity from an appropriately trained health care professional or as part of a structured educational programme.
- People with diabetes participate in annual care planning, which leads to documented agreed-on goals and an action plan.
- People with diabetes agree with their health care professional on a documented personalised HbA1c target, usually between 48 and 58 mmol/mol (6.5% and 7.5%), and receive an ongoing review of treatment to minimise hypoglycaemia.
- People with diabetes agree with their health care professional to start, review and stop medications to lower blood glucose, blood pressure and blood lipids in accordance with NICE guidance.
- Trained health care professionals initiate and manage therapy with insulin within a structured programme that includes dose titration by the person with diabetes.
- Women of childbearing age with diabetes are regularly informed of the benefits of preconception glycaemic control and of any risks, including medication that may harm an unborn child. Women with diabetes planning a pregnancy are offered preconception care, and those not planning a pregnancy are offered advice on contraception.
- People with diabetes receive an annual assessment for the risk and presence of the complications of diabetes, and these are managed appropriately.
- People with diabetes are assessed for psychological problems, which are then managed appropriately.
- People with diabetes at risk of foot ulceration receive a regular review by a foot protection team in accordance with NICE guidance.

Continued

> **Box 4.5   Quality standards set for adults with diabetes—cont'd**
>
> - People with diabetes with a foot problem requiring urgent medical attention are referred to and treated by a multidisciplinary foot care team within 24 h.
> - People with diabetes admitted to a hospital are cared for by appropriately trained staff, provided with access to a specialist diabetes team, and given the choice of self-monitoring and managing their own insulin.
> - People admitted to a hospital with diabetic ketoacidosis receive educational and psychological support prior to discharge and are followed up by a specialist diabetes team.
> - People with diabetes who have experienced hypoglycaemia requiring medical attention are referred to a specialist diabetes team.
>
> *Source: National Institute for Health and Clinical Excellence (2011a).*

Inequalities in diabetes care

Health inequalities are preventable and/or unfair differences in health status between individuals, populations or social groups. The causes of health inequalities are complex and include individual-level behavioural risk factors alongside wider determinants such as socioeconomic, environmental and cultural conditions. Socioeconomic disadvantage is associated with numerous behavioural factors that increase the risk of diabetes and its complications, but inequalities also persist in diabetes care and in the diagnosis, treatment, control and monitoring of diabetes. They may also be related to other social factors such as age, gender and ethnicity. Furthermore, gypsies and travellers, people with mental illness, prisoners, homeless people, refugees and asylum seekers and people in residential homes may also experience disadvantages in relation to diabetes care. It is thus important that accessibility and acceptability of diabetes services are maximised so that people from disadvantaged backgrounds receive the most effective care and management once diabetes is diagnosed.

A systematic review in OECD countries (ie, those above a certain level of economic development) showed that socioeconomic inequalities in the diagnosis and control of type 1 and type 2 diabetes exist even where there is universal health coverage (Ricco-Cabelli et al., 2010). A more recent review, focused mainly on type 2 diabetes, differentiated between individual-level socioeconomic status and regional deprivation, and between processes and outcomes of care, to give a more detailed picture (Grintsova et al., 2014). Surprisingly few studies have investigated associations between individual-level socioeconomic status or regional deprivation and diabetes-specific complications. However, there is consistent evidence for associations between lower individual-level socioeconomic status and process indicators (lower frequency of clinical measurements) and poorer glycaemic control (but not blood pressure or lipid levels). The associations for regional deprivation appear to be less strong for the process measures but more consistent for the intermediate outcomes. It is likely that these documented inequalities arise as the result of an interplay between individual and health care-related factors, such as regional differences in resources; this interplay is also likely to differ between individual countries. The review did not identify strong evidence for the existence of inequalities by gender in access to diabetes services. However, there was evidence for inequalities in access to diabetes services by ethnic groups, although these may be mediated by socioeconomic status (Ricco-Cabelli et al., 2010).

In the UK, a study 10 years ago highlighted inequalities relating to 17 quality-of-care indicators among 54,000 people with diabetes from 237 GPs (Hippisley-Cox et al., 2004). People from areas of high deprivation were less likely to have BMI and smoking status recorded; they were less likely to have undergone retinal screening, microalbuminuria testing, neuropathy testing and flu vaccine; and they were more likely to have high HbA1c levels and high blood pressure. Similarly, people from ethnic backgrounds were less likely to have measures recorded. The Quality and Outcomes Framework (QOF) is an annual reward and incentive programme for activity in GPs, and although there is some evidence to suggest that inequalities in diabetes care processes may have initially widened but then narrowed after the introduction of QOF (Akanuwe et al., 2010; Kontopantelis et al., 2012), there is still conflicting evidence on whether it is improving or worsening health inequalities in the UK (Dixon et al., 2010).

Patients with diabetes need to have sufficient knowledge to manage their condition effectively, as do the caregivers of children with type 1 diabetes. There is some evidence that knowledge about diabetes may be lower among people from lower socioeconomic backgrounds (Grintsova et al., 2014), but whether such inequalities are the result of differential access to structured diabetes education by social group is difficult to determine. A study in Germany suggests that participation in diabetes education programmes is lower among patients from low socioeconomic backgrounds (Mielck et al., 2006), but there is limited empirical evidence for social inequalities in access to structured diabetes education in the UK. However, in England and Wales in 2011/12 only 2% and 12% of patients newly diagnosed with type 1 and 2 diabetes, respectively, were offered access to structured education, and only around one-quarter actually took it (Diabetes UK, 2013). There are also concerns that provision varies geographically. To maximise uptake of

---

Box 4.6   Case study. Education for vulnerable people with diabetes

This Danish project is a collaboration between the Danish Diabetes Association, Patient Education Research at Steno Health Promotion Centre and the Region of Southern Denmark, who recognise that many vulnerable patients with diabetes do not take part in the diabetes education that is offered to them or are unable to translate what they learn into everyday life. These vulnerable patients often have low education, low income and low literacy skills. The project will use a Design-Thinking approach to identify the educational needs of vulnerable patients and their educators and then design new patient-centred and interactive education methods or tools and/or refine existing ones to suit their needs. These will be evaluated in a feasibility study, alongside a competence development concept for the educators of vulnerable patients. It is hoped that this innovative approach will lead to more effective education and thus improved self-management skills and behaviours among vulnerable patients with diabetes.

Source: Targeting vulnerable people with diabetes? https://steno.dk/ da%5Cpages%5Cforskere%5Cresearchprojects%5Cpatienteducation%5Ctargeting_ vulnerable_people_with_diabetes.aspx

---

education, patients themselves have raised the importance of educational provision catering for their disabilities, being suited to their cultural needs and taught in their first language (Healthcare Commission, 2006). A good example of this is a research study in Denmark that is aiming to develop tailored educational methods and tools for vulnerable patients with diabetes (see Box 4.6).

Diabetes care in developing countries

Eighty percent of people with diabetes live in developing countries. Developing countries also have high levels of undiagnosed diabetes and of impaired glucose regulation. Given that there is a trend toward development

of diabetes at a younger age in these countries, yet diagnosis is still often delayed due to poverty or lack of awareness, this set of circumstances may generate unmanageable levels of morbidity and mortality associated with diabetic complications for the future. Furthermore, rapid westernisation is accelerating the diabetes epidemic in many developing countries. However, with even developed economies struggling to cope with the diabetes epidemic, it is difficult see how developing countries will manage the delivery of high-quality care at affordable costs, given their resource constraints. Inequalities in diabetes care between developed and developing countries are therefore likely to widen in the foreseeable future.

It is recognised that the quality of diabetes care in many developing countries is suboptimal. For example, the Diab-Care Asia study in 1998 among 24,317 patients with diabetes from 230 diabetes centres in 12 Asian countries, including India and China, showed that over half of all patients did not have a recorded HbA1c measurement (Chuang et al., 2002). Venkataraman et al. (2009) provide figures from several studies on the low proportions of patients with diabetes in India who receive blood pressure checks and other investigations. Beran and Yudkin (2006) described the poor quality of care in sub-Saharan Africa and the associated low life expectancy associated with diabetes.

The International Insulin Foundation has listed 11 points that are necessary for a positive diabetes environment to enable patients with type 1 and type 2 diabetes to access high-quality care and treatment (see Box 4.7). Although the overarching issue is lack of economic resources, there are also particular circumstances relating to these 11 points that make delivery of high-quality diabetes care even more challenging in developing countries (Beran and Yudkin, 2006). There also needs to be a strong political will for diverting resources to primary prevention of diabetes.

- Health systems in many developing countries are organised primarily around the diagnosis and treatment of acute and infectious diseases. They therefore need to develop and refine

> **Box 4.7　Eleven points necessary for a positive diabetes environment**
>
> 1. Organisation of the health system
> 2. Data collection
> 3. Prevention
> 4. Diagnostic tools and infrastructure
> 5. Drug procurement and supply
> 6. Accessibility and affordability of medicines and care
> 7. Health care workers
> 8. Adherence issues
> 9. Patient education and empowerment
> 10. Community involvement and diabetes associations
> 11. Positive policy environment

capabilities for the management of chronic disease: for example, efficient systems for recall and review.
- Many health care facilities in developing countries do not currently have the resources or means to diagnose diabetes.
- Many developing countries have not yet developed the infrastructure for the systematic recording and analysis of data that is important for effective health care planning. They are behind in terms of diabetes registries, electronic clinical records and networking between clinical centres.
- Knowledge and understanding of diabetes care and management is still relatively low even among health care workers. For example, a recent review of 35 studies highlighted the general 'information poverty' of health

workers in Africa, with some of these studies specifically exploring diabetes knowledge (Pakenham-Walsh and Bukachi, 2009). In many developing countries, there are few diabetes specialists and limited numbers of dedicated nurses (if any), with very little postgraduate training in diabetes.

- Continuous availability of essential diabetes medication is fundamental to effective diabetes care. Insulin and oral hypoglycaemic agents are included on the World Health Organization's List of Essential Medicines for a basic health care system (World Health Organization, 2011b). However, results from 30 surveys in 24 low-income countries found that the median availability of glibenclamide in the public sector was 42%, and for metformin it was 16% (Gelders et al., 2006).

- The extent to which patients themselves meet costs of care at the point of delivery varies by country, but for many patients in developing countries drugs are simply not affordable. For example, nearly 3 days' wages are needed to pay for a month's treatment with metformin in Lebanon; in Uganda and Indonesia, the figure is 6 days (Gelders et al., 2006). Among 121,051 people with diabetes in 35 low- and middle-income countries, medical expenses exceeded 25% of the total household income for 11% of all respondents (Smith-Spangler et al., 2012).

- Although adherence to the diabetic regimen is a general problem among people with diabetes, this is accentuated for those on low incomes not only because of medication costs (as described earlier), but also the direct and indirect costs of other requirements for diabetes care (such as travel to clinics, purchase of appropriate footwear, access to glucometers, etc.).

- Lack of education and low levels of literacy among some people in developing countries can lead to poor health-seeking behaviour, late presentation with complications already established, and again low levels of adherence. People may also seek alternative or traditional therapies, which may either be unsafe or result in delay in access to more effective treatments. A community survey among nearly 2000 people in four provinces in Kenya found that 73% had poor knowledge about diabetes (Kiberenge et al., 2010). One study in rural India found that only half of the surveyed population (approx. 300 adults) had even heard of diabetes as a condition. There is thus a significant need to develop culturally appropriate education materials for diverse populations, many with low literacy levels (Murinarayana et al., 2010). There may also be particular barriers around encouraging people to take exercise and to lose weight in countries where obesity is seen as a sign of social status.

- Many developing countries do not have diabetes associations, and World Diabetes Day is still only recognised in around 160 countries.

Summary points

- The favoured model for diabetes care is an integrated approach to the delivery of care. MCNs provide an example of an integrated approach.
- Diabetes is a lifelong disease, with multidisciplinary care that involves an array of care processes and standards. The delivery strategy of the National Service Framework for Diabetes advocated that all people diagnosed with diabetes should be identified in an up-to-date practice-based diabetes register.
- Registries can also be used to generate core diabetes indicators for comparisons at the regional, national and international levels.
- Several sets of quality standards have been developed for diabetes care. They have been used to highlight the wide variations that exist across countries, regions and populations.
- Social inequalities persist in the diagnosis, treatment, control and monitoring of diabetes, even in developed countries and those with universal health coverage.
- The quality of diabetes care in many developing countries is suboptimal. These countries face particular challenges in delivering high-quality diabetes care, relating to organisation of the health system, lack of diagnostic facilities, poorly developed data collection systems, shortage of trained health care workers, problems with drug availability and affordability, and low levels of diabetes knowledge, awareness and adherence.

Web pages and resources

Diabetes in Scotland. http://www.diabetesinscotland. org.uk
This website is an excellent resource for health care professionals in Scotland. The page provides links to regional MCN websites. There is also a link to the SCI-DC homepage.
http://www.ecdiabetes.eu/
European Coalition for Diabetes. Diabetes in Europe. Policy Puzzle. The state we are in. Here you can find information on national policy and practice relating to diabetes in 47 European countries.
International Diabetes Federation. Global diabetes plan 2011–2012. http://www.idf.org/sites/default/files/ Global_Diabetes_Plan_Final.pdf

This document provides an excellent summary of an audit of national diabetes action plans in every country in Europe.

Further reading

Diabetes UK. Improving the delivery of adult diabetes care through integration; 2014.
The Diabetes UK report, published in October 2014, explains how adult diabetes care can be improved to achieve better outcomes for people with diabetes.
Action for diabetes; 2014.
Prepared by the Medical Directorate, NHS England, this is an essential read for all those working in diabetes care.

5 Living with diabetes

A diagnosis of diabetes can involve significant and daunting lifestyle changes. Compared with many other chronic diseases, diabetes self-management is very complex. This can make adherence very challenging. It also means that a diagnosis of diabetes can have ramifications for many areas of daily life. This chapter explores these challenges in detail.

Adherence to diabetes self-management

The World Health Organization (WHO) has defined adherence as the extent to which a person's behaviour involving taking medication, following a diet and/ or executing lifestyle changes corresponds with agreed-on recommendations from the health care provider (World Health Organization, 2003a). A patient with diabetes is expected to engage with many different aspects of a self-care regimen, including adherence to dietary and exercise recommendations, taking oral hypoglycaemic medications or insulin (as well as any other medications), self-monitoring blood glucose levels, following foot care guidelines and attending regular diabetes-related health care appointments. Furthermore, a person with diabetes will need to monitor and respond to diabetes-related symptoms.

Adherence to medication

Worldwide, WHO estimates that adherence to medication among patients suffering from chronic disease is only around 50% (World Health Organization, 2003a). Although a sample of patients with type 1 and type 2 diabetes ranked their medication as being the most important component of their diabetic treatment regimen, still only 86% reported that they were adherent to insulin all the time (Broadbent et al., 2011). Insulin adherence was only around 62–64% in a systematic review among people with type 2 diabetes (Cramer, 2004). In a study in Tayside, Scotland, adherence to insulin was measured by the proportion of days for which sufficient insulin was obtained to receive the prescribed dose, with an estimated mean value of 70%, again for people with type 2 diabetes (Donnelly et al., 2007). Another systematic review of 17 studies that included people with type 1 and type 2 diabetes found adherence to insulin ranged from 43% to 86% (Davies et al., 2013). Adherence to insulin treatment is recognised as being particularly problematic among adolescents with type 1 diabetes (Borus and Laffel, 2010). Adherence to oral hypoglycaemic agents in type 2 diabetes ranged from 36% to 93%, with estimates from prospective studies of 67–85% for the proportion of doses that were taken as prescribed (Cramer, 2004).

Improved adherence to diabetic medication is associated with improved glycaemic control (Asche et al., 2011). However, reasons for nonadherence to diabetic medications are many and varied and may include fear of side effects (particularly weight gain and hypoglycaemia), needle anxiety (for injectable therapies), inconvenience or complexity of the treatment regimen, inaccessibility to treatment and poor levels of patient knowledge about the use and importance of therapies (Nau, 2012).

In a Cochrane review of 21 studies, Vermeire et al. (2009) identified a range of interventions that have been developed to try to improve nonadherence to medication among people with type 2 diabetes. These include nurse-led interventions, home aides, diabetes education programmes, pharmacy-based interventions and interventions relating to dosage and frequency. However, this review found little robust evidence supporting the effectiveness of these interventions. This may be because there is currently no accepted theoretical model that adequately predicts and explains this kind of nonadherence. There is growing interest in new technologies such as SMS to improve adherence to insulin in young people with type 1 diabetes (Borus and Laffel, 2010).

Self-monitoring of blood glucose

Self-monitoring of blood glucose as part of an integrated care package is generally recommended for people with type 1 diabetes and for those with type 2 diabetes who are being treated with insulin. Optimal frequency may vary according to an individual's particular needs (National Institute for Clinical Excellence, 2004), although the American Diabetes Association recommends monitoring at least three times daily (American Diabetes Association, 2011). Despite this, the frequency of self-monitoring among many insulin-treated patients is lower than this. For example, a British-Danish study among over 1000 young people with type 1 diabetes found that 3% did no monitoring at all, and 61% did not test on a daily basis (Hansen et al., 2009). A study in Tayside, Scotland, found that 10% of insulin-treated patients with type 2 diabetes did no monitoring at all in 2009 (Evans et al, 2012).

Given that self-monitoring of blood glucose is associated with improved glycaemic control in insulin-treated patients, attention is turning toward interventions to improve self-monitoring. For example, Farmer et al. (2005) discussed whether telemedicine might have a role to play in enhancing the effectiveness of self-monitoring.

Foot care

People with diabetes are advised to check their feet on a daily basis to minimize the risks of developing foot ulcers. However, adherence to this recommendation is also low. For example, in an American study, 38% of a sample of 1482 people with diabetes reported never spending any time on foot care (Safford et al., 2005). In a UK study, 18.5% of people with diabetes did not inspect their feet (Pollock et al., 2004). Systematic reviews of educational interventions for improved preventive foot self-care have found only short-term benefits (Valk et al., 2001), but qualitative research suggests that some people's beliefs and practices surrounding foot care may need to be challenged more strongly (Gale et al., 2008).

Adherence to dietary and exercise recommendations

The nutritional requirements and the importance of a healthy diet for people with type 1 diabetes are similar to those for the general population, with an emphasis on fruits and vegetables, whole-grain foods and foods low in fat. In addition, though, there are the challenges of monitoring carbohydrate intake and balancing carbohydrate and insulin levels. In a narrative review of 23 studies on adherence to diet among young people with type 1 diabetes, Patton (2011) reports that adherence to dietary recommendations ranged from 21% to 95%, depending on the behaviour studied, how it was measured, and the carbohydrate regimen followed. In another study, only 22% of a mixed group of people with diabetes reported complete adherence to dietary recommendations (Broadbent et al., 2011). This is perhaps not surprising, given that participants in the same study rated diet and exercise as the least important component of their diabetic regimen.

The current recommendations for people with type 2 diabetes is that they carry out at least 150 min a week of moderate to vigorous aerobic exercise spread out over at least 3 days of the week, with no more than 2 consecutive days between exercising (Colberg et al., 2010). Regular exercise promotes weight loss and has beneficial effects on glycaemic control. However, only 17% of a mixed group of people with diabetes reported complete adherence to exercise recommendations.

Numerous lifestyle interventions for increasing physical activity and improving the diet of people with diabetes have been investigated in trials, many with moderate success. However, the challenge remains to translate these intensive interventions for incorporation into clinical practice in the 'real-world' setting, especially when people report that adhering to dietary recommendations is the most difficult aspect of diabetes self-management.

Clinic attendance

The idea of regular review of people with diabetes is explicit in many statements of diabetes care, such as the National Institute of Clinical Excellence, NICE (2011b) quality standards. In England, only 32% of people with type 1 diabetes and 52% with type 2 diabetes received all the recommended annual tests or investigations in 2009/2010 (The NHS Information Centre, 2011). However, it is almost impossible to ascertain the extent to which this is the result of patient nonattendance, which is thought to be particularly high among young people with diabetes. It is clearly important that practices have an efficient recall and review system for their diabetic patients, but patients themselves also need to understand the importance of the annual review (Box 5.1).

As with many chronic diseases, nonattendance at outpatient clinics is also a problem in diabetes care (Paterson et al., 2010). The reasons for nonattendance are complex and multifactorial and might be either health-system or patient related. A study in southeast England estimated an outpatient clinic's nonattendance rates to be around 16% in a sample of young people with type 1 diabetes (Snow and Fulop, 2012), but other studies have found the figure to be much higher. Although evidence suggests that nonattenders are more likely to have poor glycaemic control (Rhee et al., 2005), this is unlikely to reflect a simple causal association.

Box 5.1 Apps and technological solutions in diabetes

Over 90% of people in the UK now own a mobile phone. Smartphone applications ('apps') for self-management of diabetes have proliferated since 2008, when the first app was launched. A review conducted in 2013 (Arnhold et al., 2014) identified around 650 apps supported by two different platforms (some for patients, some for health care professionals), of which over half were free. The types of functions provided included documentation and/or interpretation of blood glucose values, data forwarding or communication, provision of information, recipe suggestions, a reminder function (timer) and an advisory function (therapeutic support), although over half of the apps had only one function.

Despite these many diabetes apps available, as well as a plethora of diet- and exercise-related apps relevant to people with diabetes, their potential for improving adherence to the diabetic regimen has yet to be fully realised. There seems to be no current market leader in diabetes apps, with functionality and usability needing to be improved, particularly if the apps are targeted at older people.

Source: Arnhold et al. (2014).

Living with diabetes

The WHO defines health as a state of complete physical, mental and social well-being and not merely the absence of disease or infirmity. It is therefore important to consider how diabetes can affect the social functioning of individuals within their families and communities.

Diabetes, families and social support

A diagnosis of diabetes is likely to have an effect on the family and/or friends of the individual concerned. They may need to provide emotional support to them, as well as having to deal with their own emotional reactions (such as anxiety, guilt, resentment). The changes in behaviour and lifestyle that are required may directly involve the family, particularly those surrounding diet and exercise, and friends may also need to be aware of restrictions imposed by the diabetic regimen. Furthermore, friends and family may require sufficient knowledge and understanding of diabetes to be able to assist with episodes of hypo- or hyperglycaemia.

These implications for friends and family can be conceptualised as 'social support', with most theories of behaviour change including a component for social support. There are various working definitions of social support. Social support can be regarded as a combination of structural components (social integration and the extent to which an individual is part of a social network) and functional components (transactions between individuals and perceived and actual support received). The support received can be further divided into instrumental support (tangible help or assistance) and emotional support. Social support has been shown in many different situations and conditions to be associated with improved health outcomes; the extent to which this is a direct association (the direct effect hypothesis) or whether social support simply mediates or buffers the effect of negative experiences (the buffer hypothesis) is debated.

Many studies report improved diabetes outcomes among people with higher levels of social support (Miller and DiMatteo, 2013). In terms of family, structural aspects of family (being married, living arrangements, family cohesion and organisation) are often associated with improved regimen adherence. Similarly, tangible practical and emotional support from the immediate family is associated with improved diabetes outcomes. However, there are some interesting gender differences, with men more likely to rely solely on their spouse for diabetes support, but women drawing on wider social networks. Alongside the general consensus that lack of social relationships is a risk factor for morbidity and mortality, particularly among men, wider social support has also been shown to be associated with improved diabetes-related outcomes (Kadirvelu et al., 2012).

However, there can also be barriers to self-management associated with friends and family. For example, attempts to support self-management can be perceived negatively (eg, nagging), people with diabetes report finding it more difficult to follow their diet plans when people around them are eating unhealthy foods, friends and family members may not have accurate or up-to-date knowledge and information, and they may even undermine self-management, particularly if relationships are conflicted or if they are struggling to promote independence in a child, for example. Nevertheless, there are convincing arguments for placing more emphasis on the wider social support network, in addition to patients and health care providers, in models of diabetes care.

> **! Thinking point**
>
> What advice would you give family and friends in their role of supporting someone with diabetes?

Diabetes and education

Children spend around 15,000 h at school up to the age of 16 years. Those with type 1 diabetes are likely to need additional help and support during the school day to assist them in the management of their condition. For example, they may need to self-monitor their blood glucose levels, take insulin or

other medication, eat snacks regularly, have lunch at specified times and be able to recognise and treat hypoglycaemic symptoms. Furthermore, they should not be disadvantaged in their learning or be excluded from any school or extracurricular activity. However, an online survey of 434 parents of children with type 1 diabetes found that 38% of their children did not have a care plan in school that suited their needs, and 22% were dissatisfied with the support their child received in school. In England, all schools are now required by law (from September 2014) to make sure that children with medical conditions such as type 1 diabetes get the proper care in school. In Scotland, the Education (Additional support for learning; Scotland) Act (2004) places duties on education authorities to identify, meet and keep under review the additional support needs of all pupils for whom they are responsible, including pupils with diabetes. Similarly, other educational providers also have a duty to ensure that individuals with diabetes are not discriminated against or disadvantaged.

Diabetes and adolescence

Adolescence can be a particularly difficult time for any young person as they negotiate the move from a dependent childhood to a state of independence, while maintaining a balance between freedom and responsibility. They may then leave home and adopt a more mobile and less-regulated lifestyle. Adolescent behaviours can include challenging authority, nonconformity, pleasure-seeking behaviour, heightened awareness of self-image and peer pressure. For a young person with type 1 diabetes, these behaviours have implications for diabetes self-management, and there are also hormonal and metabolic challenges to contend with. There also needs to be gradual transfer of the responsibility for diabetes self-management from the caregiver to the young person.

During puberty the body is less sensitive to insulin, requirements can increase by up to 50% and good blood glucose control is difficult to maintain. Alongside, or sometimes as a result of, this, adherence to self-management can worsen, with young people tending to focus more on short-term outcomes, whereas their caregivers and health professionals may be more concerned with longer-term outcomes. Young people with diabetes are also more at risk of depression, anxiety, low self-esteem and eating disorders (especially girls). The difficulties associated with adolescence can occur at around the time when young people are required to make the transition from paediatric to adult diabetes services, at around 16–18 years of age, depending on the location.

Over the last two decades, increasing prevalence of obesity during childhood and adolescence has resulted in diagnoses of type 2 diabetes occurring among young people (Diabetes UK, 2012a). There are currently thought to be around 500 young people with type 2 diabetes in the UK who may also face psychological and emotional problems surrounding their condition and its management.

Diabetes and employment

Under the Equality Act (2010) it is unlawful for an employer to treat a job applicant or an employee unfairly because of a disability. An employer has a duty to make reasonable adjustments to prevent a disabled employee from being placed at a substantial disadvantage in any aspect of their employment, including recruitment and selection, training, transfer, career development and retention.

For most people, a diagnosis of diabetes will not affect their employment, although the employer relies on the employee to disclose their diagnosis. The sorts of reasonable adjustments that might then be needed for an employee with diabetes include such things as having an appropriate location to store insulin or other items, having a private room available to inject insulin, being given time off to attend appointments and having regular work schedules or a predictable routine.

Some jobs may involve an element of risk and may therefore be hazardous for an employee with diabetes. There will then need to be an individual medical assessment. However, the Armed Forces is the only institution in the UK that still has a blanket ban on recruitment of people with diabetes. Other employers, such as the emergency services and the Civil Aviation Authority, have recently lifted their blanket bans, although there may still be medical requirements surrounding control of their diabetes that need to be met.

Diabetes, driving and the Driver and Vehicle Licencing Agency

Being able to drive is seen to be essential by the majority of adults; this also holds true for those with diabetes. It has proved difficult to establish whether drivers with diabetes in general have a higher risk of accidents when compared to other drivers, partly because of the difficulty in controlling for confounding in studies that are by necessity observational (Inkster and Frier, 2013). Provided that they are medically fit, however, there is no reason why people with diabetes should not be able to drive. However, hypoglycaemia has been shown to be a risk factor for driving-related mishaps (and this is reflected in the current Driver and Vehicle Licencing Agency (DVLA) regulations for drivers with diabetes).

In the UK, for Group 1 vehicles (cars and motorcycles), drivers with diabetes who are treated with insulin must inform the DVLA (unless the insulin treatment is temporary). The licence will be issued for 1, 2 or 3 years depending on their individual medical

circumstances. There is no requirement for a driver to inform the DVLA of their diabetes if they are managed by diet and/or tablets (including treatment with sulfonylureas). However, all drivers with diabetes (including those who are diet and/or tablet treated) must inform the DVLA if they:

- Experienced more than one episode of severe hypoglycaemia (requiring assistance from another person) during the previous 12-month period.
- Develop impaired awareness of hypoglycaemia.
- Experience severe hypoglycaemia when driving.
- Experience a worsening in any existing medical condition.

For Group 2 vehicles (heavy goods vehicles, HGVs, and passenger carrying vehicles, PCVs), the blanket ban on licencing people with insulin-treated diabetes was lifted in 2011. These drivers can apply for a Group 2 licence provided that they undergo annual independent medical assessments and meet strict medical criteria (no episodes of severe hypoglycaemia in the previous 12 months, full hypoglycaemic awareness and an understanding of the risk of hypoglycaemia). They must self-monitor their blood glucose regularly (at least twice daily using a glucometer with a memory function) and thus be able to demonstrate good blood glucose control for the previous 3-month period. This means it is necessary for drivers who initiate treatment with insulin to have a 3-month break from driving to accumulate the required blood glucose test results.

Diabetes and social life

For many people, eating out is an important part of their social life. However, for people with insulin-treated diabetes, it is often very difficult to determine the exact content of their meals and how to adjust insulin doses accordingly. Following simple guidelines when ordering can assist with this (see Diabetes UK, Tips for eating out). Similarly, people with type 2 diabetes should try to choose healthier options and to cut down on portion size. Despite this, many people with diabetes have learned not to let diabetes affect their ability to eat out in restaurants, at friends' houses or on social occasions. There is no need for people with diabetes to abstain from alcohol either, provided that they drink sensibly and within recommended guidelines for people with diabetes (two units for women, three units for men per day). However, alcohol does increase the risk of hypoglycaemia, and people with diabetes should avoid drinking on an empty stomach and sustained or binge drinking.

Diabetes and sex

Up to 50% of men and 25% of women may experience some kind of sexual problem or lack of desire associated with their diabetes or medication. This may be due, for example, to erectile dysfunction in men and recurrent vaginitis and cystitis in women. Although the causes of sexual dysfunction can be complex and multifaceted, maintaining good diabetes control is a first step toward addressing sexual problems.

Diabetes and travel

Although there need be no restrictions or barriers to foreign travel for people with type 1 or type 2 diabetes, they do need to take certain precautions and plan in advance. Having a doctor's letter and diabetes ID is advisable (and essential in some circumstances). In general, travellers should take at least twice as many medical supplies as they think they will need. They need to be aware that travel and holidays will necessarily mean a deviation from their usual routines, including diet and exercise, especially if crossing time zones, and that this may affect their blood glucose control. Insulin may also be absorbed faster in hot climates, so blood glucose levels need to be checked more regularly. Travellers who use insulin should find out what types and strengths of insulin are available in the area in which they will be travelling in case they run out of supplies. For storage, insulin should be kept out of direct sunlight and kept cool, but never allowed to freeze. Air travellers should therefore carry insulin and equipment in their hand luggage, for which a doctor's letter is required (Box 5.2).

! Thinking point

How might travel immunisations, the local weather and changing time zones control diabetes?

Box 5.2   Ten tips for travellers with diabetes

1. Keep your medical supplies close at hand.
2. Try to stick to your routine and adherence regimen.
3. Get documentation in case of an emergency.
4. Inform airport security you have diabetes.
5. Always be prepared to treat low glucose levels.
6. Investigate the food you eat.
7. Increase your stash of medical supplies so that you don't run out.
8. Consider time zone changes and the impact they might have on your regimen.
9. Test your blood sugar on a regular basis.
10. Tell others who you may be travelling with that you have diabetes.

Source: Joslin Diabetes Centre. www.joslin.org.

 Summary points

- Patients with diabetes are expected to adhere to many different aspects of a diabetic regimen. However, adherence remains a general problem, with more research required to identify effective interventions to improve adherence levels.
- Diabetes can have important implications for the social functioning of individuals within their families and communities, but family and friends are often a significant source of social support.
- Educational providers have a duty to ensure that individuals with diabetes are not discriminated against or disadvantaged.
- Adolescence can be a particularly difficult time for a young person with type 1 or type 2 diabetes as they negotiate the move from childhood to independence and gradually take responsibility for their own diabetes self-management. Glycaemic control can worsen during this time.
- It is unlawful for an employer to treat a job applicant or an employee unfairly because of diabetes, and reasonable adjustments may need to be made to ensure an employee with diabetes is not disadvantaged in any way.
- Provided that they are medically fit, there is no reason why people with diabetes should not be able to drive, although there will be conditions associated with their DVLA licence if they are insulin treated.
- People with diabetes should take particular care when eating out.
- Sexual dysfunction can occur in people with diabetes.
- Although there need not be restrictions or barriers to foreign travel for people with diabetes, careful planning is essential.

Web pages and resources

Diabetes and sexual activity. http://www.diabetes.co.uk/diabetes-and-sex.html.

Diet and diabetes. http://www.diabetes.org/food-and-fitness/food/what-can-i-eat/.

Employment and diabetes – an advocacy pack. http://www.diabetes.org.uk/upload/How%20we%20help/Avocacy/Employment-advocacy-pack-2013.pdf.

Noncompliance and diabetes. http://www.diabetes.org.uk/Documents/Update/Compliance[1].pdf.

Travelling and diabetes. http://www.nhs.uk/Livewell/travelhealth/Pages/travelling-with-diabetes.aspx.

Further reading

Borus JS, Laffel L. Adherence challenges in the management of type 1 diabetes in adolescents: prevention and intervention. Curr Opin Pediatr 2010;22(4):405–11.

This article reviews barriers to adherence and discusses interventions that have shown promise in improving outcomes for adolescents.

Hinder S, Greenhalgh S. "This does my head in". Ethnographic study of self-management by people with diabetes. BMC Health Services Research 2012;12:83.

This really interesting ethnographic study illustrates the challenges of self-management of diabetes in practice.

Spencer JE, Cooper HC, Milton B. The lived experiences of young people (13–16 years) with Type 1 diabetes mellitus and their parents – a qualitative phenomenological study. Diabetic Med 2013;30:e17–24.

This study provides a fascinating insight into the experiences of adolescents living with type 1 diabetes.

6 Public health prevention of diabetes

Measures to prevent disease within a population can be applied at different stages of the natural course of a disease. *Primordial prevention* seeks to prevent the emergence and establishment of risk factors for disease within a population, whether these factors are environmental, economic, social, behavioural or cultural. *Primary prevention* aims to modify risk factors once they are present in the population and to prevent individual exposure to them. *Secondary prevention* relates to measures that promote early diagnosis of a disease and associated treatment to limit its progression, with *tertiary prevention* focusing mainly on managing health problems and maximising quality of life in people with established disease.

Primordial prevention of type 2 diabetes: Population approaches to diabetes prevention

Primordial prevention of type 2 diabetes involves the prevention of diabetes-related risk factors emerging or becoming established in the population. Given that a healthy diet, regular physical activity, maintenance of a healthy weight, moderate alcohol consumption and avoidance of sedentary behaviours and smoking are all associated with reduced risk of type 2 diabetes, the promotion of environmental, economic, social, behavioural or cultural conditions that support these behaviours constitutes primordial prevention. For example, the recent smoking ban legislation in several countries illustrates the potential of population interventions to bring about behaviour change in smoking and to improve health outcomes (Callinan et al., 2010). Similarly, the proposed minimum unit pricing for alcohol in Scotland provides another example of primordial prevention, and it could have similar impact to unit pricing policy in Saskatchewan, Canada, where a 10% increase in minimum alcohol price resulted in decreased alcohol consumption (Stockwell et al., 2012).

Other potential primordial prevention initiatives for type 2 diabetes might necessitate changes in policy and environment, relating to community design, transport policy, community facilities available for recreation and leisure, the availability and cost of healthy (and unhealthy foods), food labelling, the provision of safe cycling and walking routes and physical education policies in schools. Such initiatives, whether locally or nationally implemented, often require multisectoral involvement from community-based organisations and social institutions, in a range of settings, including worksites, schools, the media or government. The National Institute for Clinical Excellence (NICE) has published guidelines on population and community interventions to prevent type 2 diabetes (National Institute for Clinical Excellence, 2011b), many of which could be defined as primordial prevention. NICE makes 10 recommendations, also emphasising the importance of culturally appropriate interventions and ensuring that healthy lifestyle messages are reaching the population. Four recommendations relate to national and local actions to promote healthy diet and physical activity. Examples of possible actions to support these recommendations are provided, and some are reproduced in Boxes 6.1 and 6.2.

 Thinking point

Would you add anything else to these prevention recommendations?

Box 6.1   Primordial prevention of type 2 diabetes through healthy diet

National action to promote a healthy diet

- Work with food manufacturers and caterers to improve the nutritional content of foods.
- Work with food manufacturers, caterers and retailers to provide clear and consistent nutrition information.
- Work with food retailers to ensure that a range of portion sizes are available and that pricing favours healthier choices.
- Support the development of home cooking.

Local action to promote a healthy diet

- Provide information on how to prepare healthy food on a budget and make people aware of their eligibility for welfare benefits schemes.
- Provide accessible nutrition education sessions.
- Work with food retailers, caterers and workplaces to encourage local provision of healthy food, with incentives to promote healthy choices.
- Encourage local caterers to provide nutritional information on menus.

Source: Adapted from NICE public health guidance 35 (NICE, 2011b).

> **Box 6.2   Primordial prevention of type 2 diabetes through increased physical activity**
>
> **National action to promote physical activity**
> - Ensure that people are aware of the benefits of physical activity.
> - Use planning regulations to maximize opportunities for people to be physically active.
> - Use planning guidance to ensure that physical activity is an objective of transport policy and the wider built environment.
>
> **Local action to promote physical activity**
> - Ensure that local planning departments support the provision of open and green spaces for walking and cycling, make local facilities and services accessible by foot and bike, and provide physical activity opportunities in safe and accessible locations.
> - Provide opportunities for activity that are affordable, practical and culturally acceptable.
> - Ensure that commissioned leisure services are affordable and acceptable.
> - Encourage local employers to develop policies to support employees to be more active (e.g. flexible working, provision of showers, secure cycle parking).
>
> *Source: Adapted from NICE public health guidance 35 (NICE, 2011b).*

Primary prevention of type 2 diabetes: Raising awareness in the population

Education and awareness are fundamental to primary prevention of disease. Increasing community understanding of a health threat such as diabetes will result in strengthened community support for the changes required for prevention. Despite the increasing prevalence of diabetes, studies from around the world indicate that knowledge and awareness of diabetes and its complications remain poor. For example, 10% of a sample of 377 British adults in 2010 could not recognise one diabetes symptom (ERS, 2011). The World Diabetes Day campaign is held annually on November 14 (the birth date of Frederick Banting) to raise global awareness of diabetes and its complications. The campaign is led by the International Diabetes Federation and its member associations around the world, including the American Diabetes Association (ADA), Diabetes UK, Diabetes Australia, the Canadian Diabetes Association, Diabetes South Africa, Diabetes New Zealand and the Diabetic Association of India. Awareness-raising activities include radio and television programmes, sporting events, public information meetings and lectures, poster and leaflet campaigns, diabetes workshops and exhibitions, press conferences, newspaper and magazine articles and many others.

Awareness-raising is paramount in the work of Diabetes UK, who have spearheaded national media awareness campaigns. For example, the Diabetes Community Champion Programme was set up to educate and raise awareness of diabetes specifically among people from Black, Asian and minority ethnic communities. Since its launch in 2010, 160 volunteer Community Champions have been trained and have attended over 200 community events to educate people about diabetes (Diabetes UK, 2012b). Similarly, Diabetes UK's annual Diabetes Week in June provides a framework for a wide range of awareness-raising activities.

Primary prevention of type 2 diabetes: Targeting risk factors

When tackling risk factors that are present in the population, there will be overlaps between specific diabetes-prevention initiatives and wider public health goals, particularly when dealing with behavioural risk factors such as diet, obesity and physical activity. The advantage of focusing more widely on the benefits of a healthy lifestyle is that this positive message has relevance for the entire population, whereas focusing specifically on diabetes prevention means that messages can be targeted to high-risk populations, as in Canada's Aboriginal Diabetes Initiative (see Box 6.3).

Obesity is one of the most important risk factors for diabetes, accounting for over 80% of the risk of developing diabetes. At the national level, the

---

Box 6.3   Case study. The Aboriginal Diabetes Initiative

The Aboriginal Diabetes Initiative (ADI) was set up in 1999 as part of the Canadian Diabetes Strategy. The goal of the ADI was to reduce type 2 diabetes among Aboriginal populations in Canada, which included 600 First Nations and Inuit communities. One of the six objectives of the ADI was 'creating supportive environments and increasing the practice of healthy behaviours through improved access to healthy food and promotion of healthy eating, physical activity, and healthy body weights'. As such, the ABI has backed several community-based prevention initiatives, such as community kitchens and gardens, healthy food box programmes, store-based education and skill development activities, and traditional food harvesting, preparation and preservation. Examples of other initiatives relating to diet and physical activity are provided on their website (see Web pages and resources).

Department of Health's strategy on obesity and Scotland's Route Map toward Health Weight describe how obesity is being tackled (Department of Health, 2012; Scottish Government, 2011). Social marketing, where the tools and techniques of marketing are used to promote behavioural change in the population, has also been used to tackle obesity; a good example being the Department of Health's Change4Life campaign (see Box 6.4). The use of financial incentives to promote healthy behaviours in the population is a controversial issue but has been implemented in the United States with some success: for example, as part of a worksite diabetes prevention weight loss programme in four nursing home facilities in Connecticut (Faghri and Li, 2014).

There is also growing interest in what is termed the 'small change' approach, whereby people are encouraged to make conscious small changes in their behaviours. The hope is that they will ultimately lead to small but significant shifts in the distribution of behavioural risk factors for diabetes at the population level. For example, Hill (2009) discusses the implications of a small-changes approach to obesity. Such

---

Box 6.4   Case study. The Change4Life campaign

The Change4Life campaign launched by the Department of Health in England in 2009 is a good example of primary prevention at the population level: a national social marketing campaign designed to address obesity in England (Department of Health, 2010). Along with Cancer Research UK and the British Heart Foundation, Diabetes UK was an early supporter of the Change4Life campaign. It was initially targeted at families with children between 5 and 11 years of age who were at high risk of overweight and obesity, with the aim of encouraging the adoption of eight 'healthy' behaviours:

- Cut back fat: reduction in fat intake, particularly saturated fat.
- Sugar swaps: reduction in intake of added sugar.
- Me size meals: control of portion size.
- Meal time: introduction of three regular meals per day.
- 5 a day: introduction of five portions of fruit and vegetables per day.
- Snack check: reduction in the number of snacks.
- 60 active minutes: at least 60 min of moderate intensity per day.
- Up and about: reduction in time spent in sedentary activity.

Change4Life relied on cross-governmental support, buy-in from NHS staff, local authorities and primary care trusts, and partnership with community and commercial organisations. Its many sub-brands, including Play4Life, Swim4Life and Walk4Life, are becoming increasingly recognised. Change4Life for adults was launched in 2010, and Start4Life is targeted at children under 5 years of age.

initiatives may at least complement individual-based population strategies but they need further evaluation.

Primary prevention of type 2 diabetes: Interventions targeted at high-risk individuals

Primary prevention at the population level can be complemented by interventions in high-risk individuals to reduce their risk of progression to type 2 diabetes. These include people with impaired glucose regulation (IGR), which has a prevalence of around 15% in adults, and those with other significant risk factors. In the absence of a formal screening programme for diabetes (see next section), the challenge is to optimise identification of these individuals so that they can benefit from targeted interventions. For example, high-risk individuals may be identified within existing anticipatory care programmes, such as the NHS Health Check Programme. This offers risk assessment to people ages 40–74 years every 5 years in England; in Scotland the Keep Well and Well North initiatives are similar. However, there are some concerns over low levels of delivery of these checks (Diabetes UK, 2012c).

NICE has published recommendations on the identification of people at high risk of diabetes outside existing programmes, and the individual level interventions that are available to them (National Institute for Clinical Excellence, 2012). NICE advocates a two-stage process. The first stage involves risk assessment using validated self-assessed questionnaires or web-based tools, with the following individuals particularly encouraged to undergo risk assessment (excluding pregnant women): all adults over 40 years; people ages 25–39 of South Asian, Chinese, African-Caribbean, Black African and other high-risk black and minority ethnic groups; and adults with conditions that increase the risk of type 2 diabetes. Self-assessment tools can be offered in a wide variety of health (community pharmacies, dental surgeries, walk-in health centres and opticians) and community venues (workplaces, job centres, leisure services, libraries, shops and faith centres) by different practitioners. Risk assessments can also be conducted by health professionals both within and outside general practice (GP), although GPs should keep a record of all risk assessment results and also actively seek out patients for risk assessment using electronic health records. Diabetes UK provides a website that enables people to complete their own diabetes risk assessment online. They are asked a series of seven questions relating to age, sex, ethnic group, whether they have relatives with diabetes, waist circumference, BMI and blood pressure; then graded as low, moderate or high risk of developing diabetes (see Web pages and resources).

NICE then recommends that people with low-risk scores should be reminded of the importance of a healthy lifestyle and encouraged to redo an assessment at least every 5 years. However, those with a high-risk score should be advised to make an appointment with their GP. This second stage of identification then involves a blood test, whether this be fasting plasma glucose (FPG) or HbA1c. The results will classify them as moderate risk (FPG < 5.5 mmol/L or HbA1c < 42 mmol/mol), high risk (FPG 5.5-6.9 mmol/L or HbA1c 42-47 mmol/mol), or possible type 2 diabetes (FPG > 7 mmol/L or HbA1c > 48 mmol/mol). People at moderate risk can be offered a brief intervention reminding them of the risks of diabetes and how to modify individual risk factors, whereas those at high risk may be candidates for an intensive lifestyle intervention to reduce risk of progression to type 2 diabetes. These people may not necessarily have FPG values that are diagnostic of impaired fasting glucose, but they should be offered further blood tests at least annually (Box 6.5).

Knowledge and education

It is important that people who are at high risk of type 2 diabetes understand the implications of this. However, it appears that many people with IGR are uncertain about their diagnosis, its consequences and its management, despite this being an excellent opportunity for education. Many

---

Box 6.5 Case study. Primary and secondary prevention by Diabetes UK

In 2012, as part of the Diabetes UK awareness-raising Measure Up campaign, Diabetes UK launched a series of healthy lifestyle roadshows, in collaboration with BUPA, which will visit nearly 100 locations across the UK (Diabetes UK, 2012c). Following the NICE (2012) recommendation as described earlier, up to 15,000 people will receive a free type 2 diabetes risk assessment and also be offered healthy lifestyle advice. Those who are identified at high risk will be referred to their GP for further diagnostic tests and interventions where appropriate. This provides an example of primary prevention.

Diabetes UK has long been concerned with the high numbers of people with undiagnosed diabetes, with their Missing Million campaign an early attempt to raise awareness of this problem. More recently, the UK-wide Silent Assassin campaign communicated key messages by posters and newspaper and consumer advertising. Its aim was also to target 500,000 people in the UK with undiagnosed diabetes with the messages that diabetes is a serious condition that is associated with devastating complications and to encourage them to make lifestyle changes (Diabetes UK, 2008). As such, the campaign is an example of secondary prevention.

people are not even aware that they have a diagnosis of IGR. For example, in 2005/2006, only 5% of people with 'prediabetes' in the United States were aware that they had the condition, rising to only 11% in 2010/2011 (Centers for Disease Control and Prevention, 2013). The WAKEUP study therefore devised key 'health alert' messages surrounding the condition for people diagnosed with IGR, and used an action research design to develop and pilot an educational package to encourage effective communication of these messages (Evans et al., 2007). The health messages needed to be clear and consistent as follows:

- IGR is a serious condition with a high risk of progressing to diabetes and heart disease.
- The good news is that these risks are preventable.
- To prevent progression, patients need to make lifestyle changes in terms of healthier eating (ideally losing weight) and increased physical activity.

At the very least, communication of these simple messages to people at high risk of type 2 diabetes or who are diagnosed with IGR (see Box 6.6) is very important, regardless of any subsequent intervention.

! Thinking point

What other pros and cons might there be for the use of the term prediabetes on patient resources?

Box 6.6   Terminology

The terms IGR and prediabetes are often used interchangeably. Although the term 'prediabetes' may be more understandable by the public, and clearly emphasizes its seriousness and association with diabetes, it has been argued that it is misleading because diagnosis of prediabetes is not inevitably followed by a diagnosis of diabetes. Despite this, it is very widely used on patient resources.

Lifestyle interventions

Once an individual has been identified as high risk for type 2 diabetes, the evidence for lifestyle interventions in preventing and/or delaying progression to type 2 diabetes is compelling. In a meta-analysis, Gillies et al. (2007) included seven trials and showed that lifestyle interventions were effective at reducing progression to type 2 diabetes among people with impaired glucose tolerance. In a Cochrane review of trials where the lifestyle intervention was based on weight loss and weight control (using behavioural interventions relating to diet and physical activity), Norris et al. (2005) showed that weight loss over 12 months was associated with a decrease in diabetes incidence among people with IGR. Perhaps the most widely known studies included in these meta-analyses are the Finnish Diabetes Prevention Study, the US Diabetes Prevention Program (DPP) and the China DaQing Diabetes Prevention Study.

The Finnish study included 522 middle-aged overweight adults with impaired glucose tolerance who were randomised to an intervention designed to reduce fat intake and to increase consumption of fibre, whole grains, vegetables and low-fat dairy products. There was a 58% reduction in diabetes incidence compared to controls over 4 years, and 43% over 7 years (Tuomilehto et al., 2001). The number needed to treat (NNT) for 1 year to prevent one case of diabetes was 22, and the NNT was five to prevent one case in 5 years. In the US DPP, 3234 mainly overweight adults with impaired glucose tolerance were randomised to an intensive weight loss intervention. Again, there was a marked decrease in diabetes incidence (Knowler et al., 2002). The NNT to prevent one case of diabetes in 3 years through lifestyle modification was 7. The Diabetes Prevention Programme Outcomes Study (DPPOS) was a continuation of the DPP trial and aimed to determine the longer-term effects of interventions to prevent diabetes (Diabetes Prevention Program Research Group, 2009). At 10-year follow-up, intensive lifestyle treatment reduced the rate of diabetes incidence by 34% compared with placebo. Results from the China Da Qing Diabetes Prevention Study showed that in a study of 577 adults with impaired glucose tolerance, those who received intensive lifestyle intervention had a 51% reduced risk of diabetes during the intervention phase,

and a 43% reduced incidence over 20 years of follow-up (Li et al., 2008b).

NICE has published detailed guidance on the delivery and content of intensive lifestyle-change programmes (National Institute for Clinical Excellence, 2012). For example, they should be delivered to groups of 10–15 people at high risk of developing type 2 diabetes, with the target community involved in their planning and design. They should be delivered by practitioners who have received externally accredited training, in a logical progression, adopting a person-centred approach. Participants should have at least 16 h of contact time, meeting at least eight times over 9–18 months. The programmes should be accessible in terms of time and location, with follow-up sessions offered at regular intervals for at least 2 years after the initial intervention period. They should provide advice, support and encouragement to help people to carry out at least 150 min of moderate-intensity physical activity per week, gradually lose weight to reach and maintain a healthy BMI, increase their dietary intake of high-fibre foods, reduce their total dietary intake of fat and eat less saturated fat. Recognised behaviour-change techniques should be used.

However, these types of lifestyle interventions are by definition intense and require commitment and motivation from patients and health care professionals. Patients are likely to require support initially when they are at the motivating stage, but this support also needs to be ongoing: for example, when they are making decisions and drawing up action plans, and then for self-regulation and maintaining any new behaviours. There is also the challenge of developing more pragmatic or real-world interventions that can be easily incorporated into clinical practice. The IMAGE project (see Box 6.7) is a European initiative that was set up in response to a need to improve diabetes information and knowledge surrounding public health strategies for prevention of type 2 diabetes; the project has led to the development of a toolkit for diabetes prevention that provides practical information and guidance on the development of appropriate interventions (Lindström et al., 2010).

There are some examples of group-based interventions for diabetes prevention that have been specifically

developed for routine clinical practice. These include the GOAL Lifestyle Implementation Trial, the PREPARE study and the Greater Green Triangle (GGT) diabetes prevention project. The GOAL Lifestyle Implementation Trial in Finland delivered six group counselling sessions to 352 middle-aged people at high risk of diabetes. Significant improvements in weight and total cholesterol were observed at 36 months (Absetz et al., 2009). The PREPARE study in the UK evaluated a group-based structured education programme, with and without individualised pedometer use, among overweight and obese individuals with impaired glucose tolerance. Improvements in glucose regulation were observed at 24 months among those randomised to the education plus pedometer group (Yates et al., 2011). The GGT diabetes prevention project in South Western Australia delivered six group sessions to 237 people at high risk of diabetes. Significant improvements in several clinical outcomes were evident at 12 months (Laatikainen et al., 2007).

However, the challenges of translating lifestyle interventions for adults at high risk of developing diabetes into routine clinical settings has been highlighted in a systematic review and meta-analysis (Cardona-Morrell et al., 2010). The review included 12 relevant studies, all showing that a variety of interventions were feasible in routine settings and most identifying encouraging weight

---

Box 6.7   Key messages from the IMAGE project

- Prevention is better than cure.
- The good news is that diabetes is preventable.
- Small changes in lifestyle mean big changes in health.
- Through joint efforts more people will be reached.
- The time to act is now.

Source: The IMAGE project (Lindström et al., 2010).

loss among individuals, but suggesting that the evidence was less convincing for other clinical outcomes, including diabetes risk reduction.

Pharmacological interventions

Given the challenges associated with lifestyle interventions, they may not necessarily be successful for everyone. However, there is now evidence that some pharmacological agents can also reduce progression to type 2 diabetes among high-risk individuals. Crandall et al. (2008) have considered the evidence for metformin, acarbose, troglitazone and rosiglitazone, and orlistat. Metformin was included in the DPP and was associated with a 31% reduction in incidence of diabetes among adults with impaired glucose tolerance. The NNT to prevent one case in 3 years using metformin was 14. In the DPPOS, after 10 years of follow-up, metformin treatment reduced diabetes incidence by 18% (Diabetes Prevention Program Research Group, 2009). Metformin use may therefore be warranted among people for whom lifestyle change has been unsuccessful. NICE (2012) recommends commencing treatment with metformin in high-risk individuals who are progressing to type 2 diabetes, despite their participation in an intensive lifestyle change programme, or in those who are unable to take part in such a programme.

Although the insulin-sensitising drugs troglitazone and rosiglitazone appear to be effective at reducing incidence of diabetes, there are some unresolved concerns over potential cardiotoxicity. Similarly, acarbose is also associated with reduction in diabetes incidence, but the frequency of gastrointestinal effects means that it is unlikely to gain widespread use. There is only limited evidence for the use of weight-loss agents, such as orlistat, in diabetes prevention, as they have not been widely used. However, NICE (2012) recommends that orlistat may be considered for adults who have a BMI of 28.0 kg/m^2 or more, who are progressing to type 2 diabetes, despite participation in an intensive lifestyle change programme or if they are unable to carry out any physical activity.

Secondary prevention of type 2 diabetes: Population screening

The aim of a population screening programme is to detect disease before the usual time of diagnosis in individuals who do not yet have signs and symptoms of the disease: 'to discover those among the apparently well who are in fact suffering from disease' (Wilson and Jungner, 1968). A formal screening programme generally involves the widespread administration of a test to the entire asymptomatic population to identify people who are at high risk and for whom earlier diagnosis is therefore likely to result in improved outcomes. People who screen positive then undergo diagnostic testing.

In their seminal paper, Wilson and Jungner (1968) suggested 10 principles that should be considered before a screening programme is implemented (see Box 6.8). Although since clarified and expanded, their original principles underpin the evaluation of most screening programmes today.

The debate over whether there should be population screening for type 2 diabetes has a long history.

Engelgau et al. (2000) discussed the evidence relating to seven questions, based on the original Wilson-Jungner criteria:

- they argued that diabetes is an important public health problem
- and that the natural history of diabetes is well understood
- diabetes has a recognized asymptomatic stage when it can be diagnosed
- and earlier treatment is likely to lead to improved outcomes
- reliable and acceptable screening tests are available, although further work would be required to identify the form and operational characteristics of the optimal screening test
- whether there is an economic justification for population screening for type 2 diabetes needs to be explored further
- as does the extent to which screening would need to be ongoing and systematic

---

Box 6.8   Wilson and Jungner's 10 principles for screening

The 10 general principles that should be considered before screening:

1. The condition sought should be an important health problem.
2. There should be an accepted treatment for patients with recognised disease.
3. Facilities for diagnosis and treatment should be available.
4. There should be a recognisable latent or early symptomatic stage.
5. There should be a suitable test or examination.
6. The test should be acceptable to the population.
7. The natural history of the condition, including development from latent to declared disease, should be adequately understood.
8. There should be an agreed-on policy on whom to treat as patients.
9. The cost of case-finding (including diagnosis and treatment of patients diagnosed) should be economically balanced in relation to possible expenditure on medical care as a whole.
10. Case-finding should be a continuing process and not a 'once and for all' project.

Source: Wilson and Jungner (1968).

However, an important evidence gap identified at a joint WHO and IDF meeting in 2003 was the lack of direct evidence available from randomised controlled trials (RCT) that earlier detection of type 2 diabetes results in improved outcomes, both clinical and psychosocial benefits for individuals and economic benefits for populations (World Health Organization, 2003b). The UK National Screening Committee has published very detailed criteria for the evaluation of screening programmes (also based on the original Wilson-Jungner principles). For type 2 diabetes, Waugh et al. (2007) showed that only a proportion of them are met. They also argued that the main failure is the lack of RCT evidence on the benefits of screening; this is also recognised by the American Diabetes Association (2003c). Since then, a cluster-randomised trial of stepwise population screening in 33 GPs in England found no reductions in all-cause, cardiovascular or diabetes-related mortality associated with being invited for screening (Simmons et al., 2012).

An alternative to mass population screening is targeted or selective screening. This is when screening is carried out only among individuals who are known to be at high risk of a particular outcome. The American Diabetes Association (2011) and Diabetes UK (2006) published guidance on which individuals should be targeted for screening for type 2 diabetes: the American Diabetes Association (2011) specified all overweight adults (BMI > 25 kg/m²) who had additional risk factors (physical inactivity, first-degree relative with diabetes, high-risk ethnic background, previous gestational diabetes or macrosomia, IGR, history of cardiovascular disease, polycystic ovary syndrome, HDL cholesterol and/or triglycerides above specified levels, clinical conditions associated with insulin resistance). The Diabetes UK (2006) criteria were very similar, with only subtle differences. However, although the implementation of targeted screening programmes in several countries does suggest that these approaches are feasible, their cost-effectiveness needs further research, particularly when the yield of new cases is relatively low (Greaves et al., 2004; Woolthius et al., 2009).

In the absence of a formal population or targeted screening programme in the UK, the identification of high-risk individuals must rely on existing anticipatory care programmes and the more opportunistic two-stage approach to risk identification as advocated by NICE (2012; described previously). The question of whether these will be sufficiently effective requires further attention (Box 6.9).

Box 6.9   Case study. Diabetes prevention in Finland

The Development Programme for the Prevention and Care of Diabetes in Finland is leading the way in diabetes prevention in the developed world. The DEHKO project took place between 2000 and 2010 and was concerned with primary prevention of type 2 diabetes, developing diabetes care and its quality, and supporting self-care among people with type 2 diabetes (DEHKO, 2010). Developed partly in response to the Finnish Diabetes Prevention Study, the primary prevention arm comprises three strategies: a population strategy promoting health at the national level and primarily targeting the risk factor of obesity, a high-risk strategy for those at increased risk of developing type 2 diabetes, and a third strategy for early diagnosis and management of the newly diagnosed (Finnish Diabetes Association, 2003). Although termed primary prevention by the Finnish Diabetes Association, these strategies could be considered as fitting nicely into the classification of primordial, primary and secondary prevention.

Population strategy

This strategy focuses on improving nutrition and increasing levels of physical activity by using a whole-population approach. Within this, interventions have been classified into those aimed at individuals, and those that are 'society-orientated measures', all of which can be regarded as primordial prevention.

Measures targeting individuals

1. Simple lifestyle counselling focusing on:
   a. Nutritional education
   b. Physical activity education concentrating on daily activity
   c. Weight-management courses and peer-support groups
   d. Counselling aimed at reducing smoking
2. Health promotion by media communication

Society-orientated measures

1. The level of expertise in physical activity and nutrition will be enhanced in primary and occupational health care.
2. The further training of health care and catering staff and nursery and school teachers will be enhanced.
3. The quality of mass catering will be improved.
4. The health education, nutritional education and physical education of children and young people will be enhanced.
5. Sports facilities serving the general population will be supported, and their numbers will be increased.
6. The range of low-fat and low-salt foods will be augmented.
7. Forms of daily physical activity will be taken into account in planning the built environment.
8. The contents and practice of health examinations will be improved.
9. Health promotion will be coordinated at national, provincial and municipal levels.

Box 6.9 Case study. Diabetes prevention in Finland–cont'd

10. Pharmacies will contribute to type 2 diabetes prevention with their own diabetes programme.
11. The cooperation of non-governmental organisations will be intensified.

High-risk strategy

The high-risk strategy involves identifying people with a particularly high risk of type 2 diabetes (primary prevention). They can be identified using the Type 2 Diabetes Risk Assessment Form, which was designed as part of the DEHKO project. This consists of 10 multiple-choice questions relating to age; BMI; waist circumference; daily physical activity; consumption of fruit, vegetables and berries; medication for high blood pressure; any previous high blood glucose levels; and any relatives with diabetes. The form takes only a few minutes to complete, can be completed over the Internet and within pharmacies, and gives an individual their probability of developing type 2 diabetes over the next 10 years. Depending on the score, the individual will receive general education and counselling or be referred for further investigation.

Early diagnosis and management strategy

The third strategy, the strategy of early diagnosis and management, is aimed primarily at people in the first 6 months after diagnosis of type 2 diabetes, when they are required to undergo a period of lifestyle management before the Social Security system in Finland reimburses medical care expenses. The aim is to ensure that all patients receive effective and multidisciplinary management.

Although it is still too early to say to what extent DEHKO will result in reduced prevalence of type 2 diabetes, it provides an excellent example of a concerted and comprehensive strategy for diabetes prevention.

Prevention of type 2 diabetes in developing countries

By 2030, 70% of people with type 2 diabetes will live in developing countries, specifically countries where national economic resources are inadequate and national health care systems are not well developed. Given these constraints, DPPs based on lifestyle modification probably offer the most potential for developing countries. Such programmes have been shown to be cost-effective, for example the DPPOS, although not necessarily cheap (Diabetes Prevention Program Research Group, 2012). The challenge therefore remains to identify low-cost strategies to identify people in developing countries who are at high risk of diabetes and then to deliver inexpensive lifestyle interventions. The International Diabetes Federation has also highlighted the importance of cultural sensitivity and to ensure that cultural beliefs are understood and addressed (Alberti et al., 2007).

Prevention of type 1 diabetes

As with type 2 diabetes, there are potentially multiple approaches to the prevention of type 1 diabetes, although there are significant challenges involved. The majority of cases of type 1 diabetes are of autoimmune origin, leading to destruction of the beta cells of the pancreas. This causes impaired insulin secretion, resulting in glucose intolerance and eventually development of symptoms and diagnosis. Known risk factors for type 1 diabetes include those of genetic origin (indicated by the close relatives of individuals diagnosed with type 1 diabetes themselves being at high risk) and of environmental origin (indicated by high proportions of newly diagnosed individuals having no family history of the disease). Suggested environmental risk factors include viral infections and several related to diet.

Targeting environmental risk factors among individuals who are known to be at high genetic risk of type 1 diabetes provides one possible avenue for primary preventative efforts. The protective effects of breastfeeding, delayed exposure to cow's milk proteins and early vitamin D supplementation in relation to type 1 diabetes could form the basis of

strategies to reduce the incidence in high-risk individuals, with trials such as TRIGR (Trial to Reduce IDDM in the Genetically At Risk) currently underway, and many more registered on TrialNet (Gregory et al., 2010).

A secondary prevention approach focuses on earlier identification and treatment of individuals who are likely to develop type 1 diabetes, before there is islet damage or abnormal immune activation. For example, it is possible to identify individuals with autoantibodies in the blood and abnormal insulin secretion, almost all of whom go on to develop type 1 diabetes. Even earlier in the disease process, the presence of beta-cell-directed antibodies in the blood may be markers for type 1 diabetes, as may be specific diabetes at-risk genes. However, the predictive values of these markers remain relatively low. Also, although the types of interventions being considered to reverse disease progression in high-risk individuals include antigen-specific interventions, antigen-nonspecific interventions and beta-cell replacement (Gregory et al., 2010), their effectiveness has not yet been demonstrated. At the moment, there is therefore no convincing rationale for a population screening programme (screening all children for autoimmune markers) or even a targeted screening programme (periodic screening for autoimmune markers of children known to be at high genetic risk) for type 1 diabetes.

Summary points

- Addressing risk factors, such as diet, obesity and physical inactivity, at the population level, is vitally important for the prevention of type 2 diabetes.
- A two-stage approach to identification of people at high risk of type 2 diabetes is recommended by NICE, consisting of risk assessment followed by blood testing for people who achieve high-risk scores.
- There is a role for pharmacological agents in diabetes prevention. The use of metformin is associated with reduction in diabetes among high-risk individuals and may be appropriate when lifestyle change has been unsuccessful.
- There is convincing evidence that lifestyle change based on weight loss and increasing levels of physical activity provides substantial reduction in type 2 diabetes risk and should be considered for all individuals at high risk of diabetes, such as those with IGR.
- There is insufficient evidence that the implementation of a population-wide screening programme for type 2 diabetes is warranted.
- Targeted screening programmes aimed at people at high risk of type 2 diabetes are feasible but whether these are cost-effective will depend on the yield of new people with diabetes.
- Given the lack of effective treatment for individuals at high risk of type 1 diabetes, there is currently no public health rationale for either population or high-risk screening.

Web pages and resources

Diabetes.co.uk: Overview of the prevention of type 2 diabetes. http://www.diabetes.co.uk/diabetes-prevention/#overview.

Diabetes UK. The Diabetes Risk Score. http://www.diabetes.org.uk/Riskscore/.

International Diabetes Federation. World Diabetes Day. http://www.idf.org/worlddiabetesday/about.

NHS choices: prevention of type 2 diabetes pages. http://www.nhs.uk/Conditions/Diabetes-type2/Pages/Prevention.aspx.

Preventing type 2 diabetes: population and community interventions. NICE public health guidance 35. http://guidance.nice.org.uk/PH35.

Preventing type 2 diabetes: risk identification and interventions for individuals at high risk. NICE public health guidance 38. http://guidance.nice.org.uk/PH38.

The Aboriginal Diabetes Initiative. http://www.hc-sc.gc.ca/fniah-spnia/diseases-maladies/diabete/index-eng.php.

The Change4Life homepage. http://www.nhs.uk/Change4Life/Pages/why-change-for-life.aspx.

The IMAGE project: improving diabetes prevention in Europe. http://www.image-project.eu/default.aspx?id=17.

The World Health Organization (WHO: information on WHO diabetes action online). http://www.who.int/diabetes/action_online/en/.

TrialNet. http://www.diabetestrialnet.org/about/index.htm.

This is an international network of researchers working in type 1 diabetes prevention.

Further reading

Alberti KG, Zimmet P, Shaw J. International Diabetes Federation: a consensus on type 2 diabetes prevention. Diabet Med 2007;24(5):451–63.

Goyder E, Simmons R, Gillett M. Who can prevent diabetes? Current issues in the prevention of type 2 diabetes. J R Coll Physicians Edinb 2010;40:5–11.

These two very accessible articles discuss key issues surrounding diabetes prevention.

Lindstrom J, on behalf of the IMAGE Study Group, et al. Take action to prevent diabetes in Europe. The IMAGE toolkit for the prevention of diabetes in Europe. Horm Metab Res 2010;42(Suppl. 1):S37–55.

This article gives an account of the purpose, development and content of the IMAGE toolkit for diabetes prevention.

Yates T, Davies M, Khunti K. Preventing type 2 diabetes: can we make the evidence work? Postgrad Med J 2009;85:475–80.

This article highlights findings from diabetes-prevention programmes and challenges involved in translating research into practice.

References

Absetz P, Oldenburg B, Hankonen N, Valve R, Heinonen H, Nissinen A, et al. Type 2 diabetes prevention in the "real world": three-year results of the GOAL lifestyle implementation trial. Diabetes Care 2009;32:1418–20.

Adler AI. Effectiveness of individual-level interventions to prevent vascular complications. In: Narayan KMV, Williams D, Gregg EW, Cowie CC, editors. Diabetes public health. From data to policy. USA: Oxford University Press; 2011.

Akanuwe J, Goyder E, O'Hara R, Julious S. P05 exploring the impact of the quality and outcomes framework on the quality of diabetes care and health care inequalities in England. J Epidemiol Community Health 2010;64:A35.

Alberti KGMM, Zimmet P, Shaw J. International Diabetes Federation: a consensus on type 2 diabetes prevention. Diabet Med 2007;24:451–63.

American Diabetes Association. Implications of the United Kingdom Prospective Diabetes Study. Diabetes Care 2002;25:528–32.

American Diabetes Association. Gestational diabetes mellitus. Diabetes Care 2003a;23:S103–5.

American Diabetes Association. Peripheral arterial disease in people with diabetes. Diabetes Care 2003b;26:3333–41.

American Diabetes Association. Screening for type 2 diabetes. Diabetes Care 2003c;26(Suppl. 1):S21–4.

American Diabetes Association. Standards of medical care in diabetes—2011. Diabetes Care 2011;34 (Suppl 1):S11–S16.

American Heart Association. AHA statistical update. Heart disease and stroke statistics—2012 update. A report from the American Heart Association. Circulation 2012;125:e2–220.

Arnhold M, Quade M, Kirch W. Mobile applications for diabetics: a systematic review and expert-based usability evaluation considering the special requirements of diabetes patients age 50 years or older. J Med Internet Res 2014;16:4.

Asao K, Sarti C, Forsen T, Hyttinen V, Nishimura R, Matsushima M, et al. Long-term mortality in nationwide cohorts of childhood-onset type 1 diabetes in Japan and Finland. Diabetes Care 2003;23:2037–42.

Asche C, LaFleur J, Conner C. A review of diabetes treatment adherence and the association with clinical and economic outcomes. Clin Ther 2011;33:74–109.

Barker DJP. The fetal origins of type 2 diabetes mellitus. Ann Intern Med 1999;130:322–4.

Barnett KN, Ogston SA, McMurdo MET, Morris AD, Evans JMM. A 12-year follow-up study of all-cause and cardiovascular mortality among 10,532 people newly diagnosed with type 2 diabetes in Tayside, Scotland. Diabetic Medicine 2010;27:1124–9.

Bellamy L, Casas JP, Hingorani AD, Williams D. Type 2 diabetes mellitus after gestational diabetes: a systematic review and meta-analysis. Lancet 2009;373:1773–9.

Beran D, Yudkin JS. Diabetes care in sub-Saharan Africa. Lancet 2006;368:1689–95.

Bertoni AG, Goff DC. Diabetes and cardiovascular disease. In: Narayan KMV, Williams D, Gregg EW, Cowie CC, editors. Diabetes public health. From data to policy. USA: Oxford University Press; 2011.

Boden-Albala B, Cammack S, Chong J, Wang C, Wright C, Rundek T, et al. Diabetes, fasting glucose levels, and risk of ischemic stroke and vascular events: findings from the Northern Manhattan Study (NOMAS). Diabetes Care 2008;31:1132–7.

Bonovas S, Peponis V, Filioussi K. Diabetes mellitus as a risk factor for primary open-angle glaucoma: a meta-analysis. Diabet Med 2004;21:609–14.

Borus JS, Laffel L. Adherence challenges in the management of type 1 diabetes in adolescents: prevention and intervention. Curr Opin Pediatr 2010;22:405–11.

Boulton AJM, Bowling FL. Diabetes and lower-extremity disease. In: Narayan KMV, Williams D, Gregg EW, Cowie CC, editors. Diabetes public

References

health. From data to policy. USA: Oxford University Press; 2011.

Boussageon R, Bejan-Angoulvant T, Saadatian-Elahi M, Lafont S, Kassai B, Erpeldinger S, et al. Effect of intensive glucose lowering treatment on all cause mortality, cardiovascular death, and microvascular events in type 2 diabetes: meta-analysis of randomised controlled trials. Br Med J 2012;343:d4169.

Broadbent E, Donkin L, Stroh JC. Illness and treatment perceptions are associated with adherence to medications, diet, and exercise in diabetic patients. Diabetes Care 2011;34:338–40.

Callaghan BC, Little AA, Feldman EL, Hughes RA. Enhanced glucose control for preventing and treating diabetic neuropathy. Cochrane Syst Rev 2012;13:CD007543.

Callinan JE, Clarke A, Doherty K, Kelleher C. Legislative smoking bans for reducing secondhand smoke exposure, smoking prevalence and tobacco consumption. Cochrane Database Syst Rev 2010;14:CD005992.

Cardona-Morrell M, Rychetnik L, Morrell SL, Espinel PT, Bauman A. Reduction of diabetes risk in routine clinical practice: are physical activity and nutrition interventions feasible and are the outcomes from reference trials replicable? A systematic review and meta-analysis. BMC Public Health 2010;10:653.

Centers for Disease Control and Prevention. Awareness of prediabetes—United States, 2005–2010. Morb Mortal Wkly Rep 2013;62:209–12.

Centers for Disease Control and Prevention. National diabetes statistics report, 2014; 2014. http://www.cdc.gov/diabetes/pubs/statsreport14/national-diabetes-report-web.pdf.

Chamnan P, Simmons RK, Sharp SJ, Griffin SJ, Wareham NJ. Cardiovascular risk assessment scores for people with diabetes: a systematic review. Diabetologia 2009;52:2001–14.

Cheng WS, Wingard DL, Kritz-Silverstein D, Barrett-Connor E. As good as it gets? Sensitivity and specificity of death certificates for diabetes: the Rancho Bernardo. Ann Epidemiol 2005;15:642.

Chitaley K, Kupelian V, Subak L, Wessells H. Diabetes, obesity and erectile dysfunction: field overview and research priorities. J Urol 2009;182:S45–50.

Chuang L-M, Tsai ST, Huang BY, Tai TY. The status of diabetes control in Asia—a cross-sectional survey of 24 317 patients with diabetes mellitus in 1998. Diabet Med 2002;19:978–85.

Colberg SR, Sigal RJ, Fernhall B, Regensteiner JG, Blissmer BJ, Rubin RR, et al. Exercise and type 2 diabetes. The American College of Sports Medicine and the American Diabetes Association: joint position statement. Diabetes Care 2010;33:e147–67.

Colhoun HM and the SDRN Epidemiology Group. Use of insulin glargine and cancer incidence in Scotland: a study from the Scottish Diabetes Research Network Epidemiology Group. Diabetologia 2009;52:1755–65.

Conget I, Gimenez M. Glucose control and cardiovascular disease. Is it important? No. Diabetes Care 2009;32(Suppl. 2):S334–6.

Correa-Villasenor A, Marcinkevage JA. In: Narayan KMV, Williams D, Gregg EW, Cowie CC, editors. Diabetes public health. From data to policy. USA: Oxford University Press; 2011.

Corrigan P, Grummit J, Lucas S. Integrated GP led diabetes care in Bexley; 2012. http://www.rightcare.nhs.uk/downloads/RC_Casebook_Bexley_Diabetes_Care_final.pdf.

Cramer JA. A systematic review of adherence with medications for diabetes. Diabetes Care 2004;27:1218–24.

Crandall JP, Knowler WC, Kahn SE, Marrero D, Florez JC, Bray GA, et al. The prevention of type 2 diabetes. Nat Clin Pract Endocrinol Metab 2008;4:382–93.

Cukierman T, Gerstein HC, Williamson JD. Cognitive decline and dementia in diabetes—systematic overview of prospective observational studies. Diabetologia 2005;48:2460–9.

Davies MJ, Gagliardino JJ, Gray LJ, Khunti K, Mohan V, Hughes R. Real-world factors affecting adherence to insulin therapy in patients with Type 1 or Type 2 diabetes mellitus: a systematic review. Diabetic Med 2013;30:512–24.

DEHKO. DEHKO 2003–2010; 2010. http://www.diabetes.fi/files/1101/eDehkokaavio.jpg.

Department of Health. National service framework for diabetes: delivery strategy; 2002. http://www.dh.gov.uk/prod_consum_dh/groups/dh_digitalassets/@dh/@en/documents/digitalasset/dh_4058937.pdf.

Department of Health. Change4Life: eat well, move more, live longer; 2009. http://webarchive.nationalarchives.gov.uk/+/www.dh.gov.uk/en/MediaCentre/Currentcampaigns/Change4Life/index.htm.

Department of Health. Change4Life. One year on; 2010. www.dh.gov.uk/publications.

Department of Health. An update on the government's approach to tackling obesity; 2012. http://www.nao.org.uk/wp-content/uploads/2012/07/tackling_obesity_update.pdf.

Diabetes Control and Complications Trial (DCCT) Research Group. The effect of intensive treatment of diabetes on the development and progression of long-term complications in insulin-dependent diabetes mellitus. N Engl J Med 1993;329:977–86.

Diabetes Prevention Program Research Group. 10-year follow-up of diabetes incidence and weight loss in the Diabetes Prevention Program Outcomes Study. Lancet 2009;374:1677–86.

Diabetes Prevention Program Research Group. The 10-year cost-effectiveness of lifestyle intervention or metformin for diabetes prevention: an intent-to-treat analysis of the DPP/DPPOS. Diabetes Care 2012;35:723–30.

Diabetes UK. Position statement. Early identification of people with type 2 diabetes; 2006.

Diabetes UK, et al. Joint Position Statement. Integrated care in the reforming NHS - ensuring access to high quality care for all people with diabetes; 2007. https://www.diabetologists. org.uk/Shared_documents/notice_board/ joint_statement_v4.pdf.

Diabetes UK. Diabetes. Beware the silent assassin. A report from Diabetes UK; 2008. http://www. diabetes.org.uk/Documents/Reports/Silent_ assassin_press_report.pdf.

Diabetes UK. Diabetes in the UK 2011/2012: key statistics on diabetes; 2012a. http://www. diabetes.org.uk/Documents/Reports/Diabetes-in-the-UK-2011-12.pdf.

Diabetes UK. Diabetes UK community champions; 2012b. http://www.diabetes.org.uk/Get_involved/ Raising-awareness/Community-Champions/.

Diabetes UK. Warning about the one in 70 people who have undiagnosed type 2 diabetes; 2012c. http:// www.diabetes.org.uk/About_us/News_Landing_ Page/Warning-about-the-one-in-70-people-who-have-undiagnosed-diabetes/.

Diabetes UK. State of the nation; 2013. http:// www.diabetes.org.uk/Documents/About%20Us/ What%20we%20say/0160b-state-nation-2013-england-1213.pdf.

Diabetes UK. Position statement. Diabetes specialist nurses. Improving patient outcomes and reducing costs; 2014. https://www.diabetes. org.uk/Documents/Position%20statements/ Diabetes-Specialist-Nurses_Improving-patient-outcomes-and-reducing-costs-position-statement-February2014.pdf.

DIAMOND Project Group. Incidence and trends of childhood type 1 diabetes worldwide 1990–1999. Diabet Med 2006;23:857–66.

Dixon A, Khachatryan A, Wallace A, Peckham S, Boyce T, Gillam S. The quality and outcomes framework: does it reduce health inequalities? Final report. NIHR Service Delivery and Organisation programme; 2010.

Donnelly LA, Morris AD, Evans JMM. Adherence to insulin treatment and its association with glycaemic control in patients with type 2 diabetes. Q J Med 2007;100:345–50.

Egede LE, Ellis C. Diabetes and depression: global perspectives. Diabetes Res Clin Pract 2010;87:302–31.

Engelgau MM, Narayan KMV, Herman WH. Screening for type 2 diabetes. Diabetes Care 2000;23:1563–80.

ERS. Public awareness of the symptoms of diabetes. Research report; 2011. www.e-r-s.org.uk/download. php?pageid=33.

EUBIROD. EUropean Best Information through Regional Outcomes in Diabetes; 2012. http://www. eubirod.eu/.

EURODIAB ACE Study Group. Variation and trends in incidence of childhood diabetes in Europe. Lancet 2000;355:873–6.

Evans JMM, Newton RW, Ruta DA, MacDonald TM, Morris AD. Socio-economic status, obesity and prevalence of Type 1 and Type 2 diabetes mellitus. Diabet Med 2000;17:478–80.

Evans PH, Greaves C, Winder R, Fearn-Smith J, Campbell JL. Development of an educational 'toolkit' for health professionals and their patients with prediabetes: the WAKEUP study (Ways of Addressing Knowledge Education and Understanding in Pre-diabetes). Diabet Med 2007;24:770–7.

Evans JMM, Barnett KN, McMurdo MET, Morris AD. Reporting of diabetes on death certificates of 1,872 people with type 2 diabetes in Tayside, Scotland. Eur J Pub Health 2008;18:201–3.

Evans JMM, Mackison D, Emslie-Smith A, Lawton J. Self-monitoring of blood glucose in type 2 diabetes: Cross-sectional analyses in 1993, 1999 and 2009. Diabetic Medicine 2012;29:1–4.

Faghri PD, Li R. Effectiveness of financial incentives in a worksite diabetes prevention program. Open Obes J 2014;6:1–12.

Fagot-Campagna A, Narayan KMV, Imperatore G. Type 2 diabetes in children. Br Med J 2001;322:377–8.

Farmer A, Gibson OJ, Tarassenko L, Neil A. A systematic review of telemedicine interventions to support blood glucose self-monitoring in diabetes. Diabet Med 2005;22:1372–8.

Ferrara A. Increasing prevalence of gestational diabetes mellitus. A public health perspective. Diabetes Care 2007;30(Suppl. 2):S141–6.

Finnish Diabetes Association. Programme for the prevention of type 2 diabetes in Finland; 2003. http://www.diabetes.fi/files/1108/

References

Programme_for_the_Prevention_of_Type_2_Diabetes_in_Finland_2003-2010.pdf.

Fleming BB, Greenfield S, Engelgau MM, Pogach LM, Clauser SB, Parrott MA. The diabetes quality improvement project. Diabetes Care 2001;24:1815–20.

Fox CS, Pencina MJ, Meigs JB, Vasan RS, Levitsky YS, D'Agostino RB. Trends in the incidence of type 2 diabetes mellitus from the 1970s to the 1990s. The Framingham Heart Study. Circulation 2006;113:2914–8.

Gaede P, Vedel P, Parving H-H, Pedersen O. Intensified multifactorial intervention in patients with type 2 diabetes mellitus and microalbuminuria: the Steno type 2 randomised study. Lancet 1999;353:617–22.

Gale L, Vedhara K, Searle A, Kemple T, Campbell R. Patients' perspectives on foot complications in type 2 diabetes: a qualitative study. Br J Gen Pract 2008;58:555–63.

Gelders S, Ewen M, Noguchi N, Laing R. Price, availability and affordability. An international comparison of chronic disease medicines. Geneva: World Health Organization, Health Action International; 2006.

Gillies CL, Abrams KR, Lambert PC, Cooper NJ, Sutton AJ, Hsu RT, et al. Pharmacological and lifestyle interventions to prevent or delay type 2 diabetes in people with impaired glucose tolerance: systematic review and meta-analysis. Br Med J 2007;334:299.

Greaves CJ, Stead JW, Hattersley AT, Ewings P, Brown P, Evans PH. A simple pragmatic system for detecting new cases of type 2 diabetes and impaired fasting glycaemia in primary care. Fam Pract 2004;21:57–62.

Greene A, Pagliari C, Cunningham S, Donnan P, Evans J, Emslie-Smith A, et al. Do managed clinical networks improve quality of diabetes care? Evidence from a retrospective mixed methods evaluation. Qual Saf Health Care 2009;18:456–61.

Gregg EW, Beckles GL, Williamson DF, Leveille SG, Langlois JA, Engelgau MM, et al. Diabetes and physical disability among older US adults. Diabetes Care 2000;23:1272–7.

Gregory JM, Lilley JS, Misfeldt AA, Buscariollo DL, Russell WE, Moore DJ. Incorporating type 1 diabetes prevention into clinical practice. Clin Diabetes 2010;28:61–70.

Grintsova O, Maier W, Mielck A. Inequalities in health care among patients with type 2 diabetes by individual socio-economic status (SES) and regional deprivation: a systematic literature review. Int J Equity Health 2014;13:14.

Gross JL, de Azevedo MJ, Silveiro SP, Canani LH, Caramori ML, Zelmanovitz T. Diabetic nephropathy: diagnosis, prevention, and treatment. Diabetes Care 2005;28:176–88.

Hansen MV, Pedersen-Bjergaard U, Heller SR, Wallace TM, Rasmussen AK, Jørgensen HV, et al. Frequency and motives of blood glucose self-monitoring in type 1 diabetes. Diabetes Res Clin Pract 2009;85:183–8.

Harati H, Hadaegh F, Saadat N, Azizi F. Population-based incidence of Type 2 diabetes and its associated risk factors: results from a six-year cohort study in Iran. BMC Public Health 2009;9:186.

Harrison TA, Hindorff LA, Kim H, Wines RCM, Bowen DJ, McGrath BB, et al. Family history of diabetes as a public health tool. Am J Prev Med 2003;24:152–9.

Health Survey for England. Health survey for England 2004: health of ethnic minorities—full report; 2004. http://www.ic.nhs.uk/pubs/hse04ethnic.

Healthcare Commission. The views of people with diabetes. Key findings from the 2006 survey; 2006.

Heller SRon behalf of the ADVANCE Trial. A summary of the ADVANCE trial. Diabetes Care 2009;32(Suppl. 2):S357–61.

Hex N, Bartlett C, Wright D, Taylor M, Varley D. Estimating the current and future costs of Type 1 and Type 2 diabetes in the UK, including direct health costs and indirect societal and productivity costs. Diabet Med 2012;29:855–62. http://dx.doi.org/10.1111/j.1464-5491.2012.03698.x.

Hill JO. Can a small-changes approach help address the obesity epidemic? A report of the Joint Task Force of the American Society for Nutrition, Institute of Food Technologists, and International Food Information Council. Am J Clin Nutr 2009;89:477–84.

Hippisley-Cox J, O'Hanlon S, Coupland C. Association of deprivation, ethnicity, and sex with quality indicators for diabetes: population based survey of 53 000 patients in primary care. Br Med J 2004;329:1267–70.

Hopkins D, Lawrence I, Mansell P, Thompson G, Amiel S, Campbell M, et al. Improved biomedical and psychological outcomes 1 year after structured education in flexible insulin therapy for people with type 1 diabetes: the U.K. DAFNE experience. Diabetes Care 2012;35:1638–42.

Hsu C-C, Lee C-H, Wahlqvist ML, Huang H-L, Chang H-Y, Chen L, et al. Poverty increases type 2 diabetes incidence and inequality of care despite universal health coverage. Diabetes Care 2012;35:2286–92.

Hunt KJ, Schuller KL. The increasing prevalence of diabetes in pregnancy. Obstet Gynecol Clin North Am 2007;34:173-vii.

Icks A, Haastert B, Trautner C, Giani G, Glaeske G, Hoffmann F. Incidence of lower-limb amputations in the diabetic compared to the non-diabetic population. Findings from nationwide insurance data, Germany, 2005–2007. Exp Clin Endocrinol Diabetes 2009;117:500–4.

Inkster B, Frier BM. Diabetes and driving. Diabetes Obes Metab 2013;15:775–83.

International Diabetes Federation. The IDF consensus worldwide definition of the metabolic syndrome; 2006a. http://www.idf.org/webdata/docs/IDF_Meta_def_final.pdf.

International Diabetes Federation. IDF Diabetes Atlas, 3rd edn. Brussels, Belgium: International Diabetes Federation; 2006b. http://www.idf.org/sites/default/files/Diabetes-Atlas-3rd-edition.pdf.

International Diabetes Federation, Europe. Diabetes—the policy puzzle. Is Europe making progress? 2011.

International Diabetes Federation. IDF Diabetes Atlas, 6th edn. Brussels, Belgium: International Diabetes Federation; 2013. http://www.idf.org/diabetesatlas.

Janghorbani M, Jones RB, Allison SP. Incidence of and risk factors for cataract among diabetes clinic attenders. Ophthalmic Epidemiol 2000;7:13–25.

Jeon CY, Murray MB. Diabetes mellitus increases the risk of active tuberculosis: a systematic review of 13 observational studies. PLoS Med 2008;5:e152.

Kadirvelu A, Sadasivan S, Ng SH. Social support in type II diabetes care: a case of too little, too late. Diabetes Metab Syndr Obes 2012;5:407–17.

Kiberenge MW, Ndegwa ZM, Njenga EW, Muchemi EW. Knowledge, attitude and practices related to diabetes among community members in four provinces in Kenya: a cross-sectional study. Pan Afr Med J 2010;7:2.

Kim C, Newton KM, Knopp RH. Gestational diabetes and the incidence of type 2 diabetes. A systematic review. Diabetes Care 2002;25:1862–8.

Kitabchi AE, Umpierrez GE, Murphy MB, Barrett EJ, Kreisberg RA, Malone JI, et al. Management of hyperglycemic crises in patients with diabetes. Diabetes Care 2001;24:131–53.

Kitabchi AE, Umpierrez GE, Murphy MB, Kriesberg RA. Hyperglycemic crises in adult patients with diabetes: a consensus statement from the American Diabetes Association (Consensus Statement). Diabetes Care 2006;29:2739–48.

Klein BE, Klein R, Moss SE. Incidence of cataract surgery in the Wisconsin Epidemiologic Study of Diabetic Retinopathy. Am J Ophthalmol 1995;119:295–300.

Klein R, Saaddine JB, Klein BEK. Diabetes and vision. In: Narayan KMV, Williams D, Gregg EW, Cowie CC, editors. Diabetes public health. From data to policy. USA: Oxford University Press; 2011.

Knowler WC, Barrett-Connor E, Fowler SE, Hamman RF, Lachin JM, Walker EA, et al. Reduction in the incidence of type 2 diabetes with lifestyle intervention or metformin. N Engl J Med 2002;346:393–403.

Koev DJ, Tankova TI, Kozlowski PG. Effect of structured group education on glycemic control and hypoglycemia in insulin-treated patients. Diabetes Care 2003;26:251.

Kontopantelis E, Reeves D, Valderas JM, Campbell S, Doran T. Recorded quality of primary care for patients with diabetes in England before and after the introduction of a financial incentive scheme: a longitudinal observational study. BMJ Qual Saf 2012;22:53–64. http://dx.doi.org/10.1136/bmjqs-2012-001033.

Laatikainen T, Dunbar JA, Chapman A, Kilkkinen A, Vartiainen E, Heistaro S, et al. Prevention of type 2 diabetes by lifestyle intervention in an Australian primary health care setting: Greater Green Triangle (GGT) Diabetes Prevention Project. BMC Public Health 2007;7:249.

Lancet. The global challenge of diabetes. Lancet 2008;371(9626):1723.

Lawrence JM, Contreras R, Chen W, Sacks DA. Trends in the prevalence of preexisting diabetes and gestational diabetes mellitus among a racially/ethnically diverse population of pregnant women, 1999–2005. Diabetes Care 2008;31:899–904.

Leese GP, Boyle P, Feng Z, Emslie-Smith A, Ellis JD. Screening uptake in a well-established diabetic retinopathy screening program. The role of geographical access and deprivation. Diabetes Care 2008;31:2131–5.

Li C, Ford ES, Strine TW, Mokdad AH. Prevalence of depression among U.S. adults with diabetes: findings from the 2006 behavioral risk factor surveillance system. Diabetes Care 2008a;31:105–7.

Li G, Zhang P, Wang J, Gregg EW, Yang W, Gong Q, et al. The long-term effect of lifestyle interventions to prevent diabetes in the China Da Qing Diabetes Prevention Study: a 20-year follow-up study. Lancet 2008b;24:1783–9.

Libman IM, LaPorte RE, Libman AM. Non-type 2 diabetes. Prevalence, incidence and risk factors. In: Narayan KMV, Williams D, Gregg EW, Cowie CC, editors. Diabetes public health. From data to policy. USA: Oxford University Press; 2011.

Lindström J, Neumann A, Sheppard KE, Gilis-Januszewska A, Greaves CJ, Handke U, et al. Take action to prevent diabetes—the IMAGE toolkit for the prevention of type 2 diabetes in Europe. Horm Metab Res 2010;42(Suppl. 1):S37–55.

Maahs DM, West NA, Lawrence JM, Mayer-Davis EJ. Epidemiology of type 1 diabetes. Endocrinol Metab Clin North Am 2010;39:481–97.

Masso Gonzalez EL, Johansson S, Wallander M-A, Garcia Rodriguez LA. Trends in the incidence and prevalence of diabetes in the UK 1996–2005. J Epidemiol Community Health 2009;63:332–6.

Mayer-Davis EJ, Dabelea D, Lawrence JM, Meigs JB, Teff K. Risk factors for type 2 and gestational diabetes. In: Narayan KMV, Williams D, Gregg EW, Cowie CC, editors. Diabetes public health. From data to policy. USA: Oxford University Press; 2011.

Mayne D, Stout NR, Aspray TJ. Diabetes, falls and fractures. Age Ageing 2010;39:522–5.

Mbanya JCN, Motala AA, Sobngwi E, Assah FK, Enoru ST. Diabetes in sub-Saharan Africa. Lancet 2010;375:2254–66.

McEwen LN, Karter AJ, Curb JD, Marrero DG, Crosson JC, Herman WH. Temporal trends in recording of diabetes on death certificates. Results from Translating Research Into Action for Diabetes (TRIAD). Diabetes Care 2011;34:1529–2534.

Meigs JB. Epidemiology of type 2 diabetes and cardiovascular disease: translation from population to prevention. Diabetes Care 2010;33:1865–71.

Mielck A, Reitmier P, Rathmann W. Knowledge about diabetes and participation in diabetes training courses: the need for improving health care for diabetes patients with low SES. Exp Clin Endocrinol Diabetes 2006;114:240–8.

Miller TA, DiMatteo MR. Importance of family/social support and impact on adherence to diabetic therapy. Diabetes Metab Syndr Obes 2013;6:421–6.

Minassian D, Reidy A. A report prepared for RNIB. Future sight loss UK (2): an epidemiological and economic model for sight loss in the decade 2010–2020; 2009. http://www.rnib.org.uk/aboutus/Research/reports/2009andearlier/FSUK_2.pdf.

Morris AD, Boyle DIR, MacAlpine R, Emslie-Smith A, Jung RT, Newton RW, et al. The diabetes audit and research in Tayside Scotland (DARTS) study: electronic record-linkage to create a diabetes register. Br Med J 1997;315:524–8.

Morrish NJ, Wang SL, Stevens LK, Fuller JH, Keen H. Mortality and causes of death in the WHO Multinational Study of vascular disease in diabetes. Diabetologia 2001;44(Suppl. 2):S14–21.

Mulnier HE, Seaman HE, Raleigh VS, Soedamah-Muthu SS, Colhoun HM, Lawrenson RA, et al. Risk of stroke in people with type 2 diabetes in the UK: a study using the General Practice Research Database. Diabetologia 2006a;49:2859–65.

Mulnier HE, Seaman HE, Raleigh VS, Soedamah-Muthu SS, Colhoun HM, Lawrenson RA. Mortality in people with type 2 diabetes in the UK. Diabet Med 2006b;23:516–21.

Mulnier HE, Seaman HE, Raleigh VS, Soedamah-Muthu SS, Colhoun HM, Lawrenson RA, et al. Risk of myocardial infarction in men and women with type 2 diabetes in the UK: a cohort study using the General Practice Research Database. Diabetologia 2008;51:1631–45.

Murinarayana C, Balachandra G, Hiremath SG, Iyengar K, Anil NS. Prevalence and awareness regarding diabetes mellitus in rural Tamaka, Kolar. Int J Diabetes Dev Cries 2010;30:18–21.

Nathan DM, Davidson MB, DeFronzo RA, Heine RJ, Henry RR, Pratley R, et al. Impaired fasting glucose and impaired glucose tolerance. Diabetes Care 2007;30:753–9.

National Audit Office. The management of adult diabetes services in the NHS; 2012.

National Diabetes Retinopathy Screening; 2012. http://www.ndrs.scot.nhs.uk/.

National Institute for Clinical Excellence. Clinical guideline 15. Type 1 diabetes: diagnosis and management of type 1 diabetes in children, young people and adults. London: National Institute for Clinical Excellence; 2004.

National Institute for Clinical Excellence. Clinical guideline 63. Diabetes in pregnancy. Management of diabetes and diabetic complications from pre-conception to the postnatal period; 2015. https://www.nice.org.uk/guidance/ng3.

National Institute for Clinical Excellence. Clinical guideline 87. Type 2 diabetes: the management of type 2 diabetes. London: National Institute for Clinical Excellence; 2009.

National Institute for Clinical Excellence. NICE quality standard QS06. Diabetes in adults. London: National Institute for Clinical Excellence; 2011a.

National Institute for Clinical Excellence. NICE public health guidance 35. Preventing type 2 diabetes: population and community interventions. London: National Institute for Clinical Excellence; 2011b.

National Institute for Clinical Excellence. NICE public health guidance PH38. Preventing type 2 diabetes: risk identification and interventions for individuals at high risk. London: National Institute for Clinical Excellence; 2012.

Nau DP. Recommendations for improving adherence to type 2 diabetes mellitus therapy—focus on optimizing oral and non-insulin therapies. Am J Manag Care 2012;18:S49–54.

Newman-Casey PA, Talwar N, Nan B, Musch DC, Stein D. The relationship between components of metabolic syndrome and open-angle glaucoma. Ophthalmology 2011;118:1318–26.

NHS Diabetes. Commissioning diabetes without walls; 2009. http://www.yearofcare.co.uk/sites/default/files/images/diabeteswithoutwalls1.pdf.

NHS Diabetic Eye Screening Programme; 2012. http://diabeticeye.screening.nhs.uk/statistics.

Nichols GA, Gullion CM, Koro CE, Ephross SA, Brown JB. The incidence of congestive heart failure in type 2 diabetes. Diabetes Care 2004;27:1879–84.

Nield L, Moore HJ, Cruickshank K, Hooper L, Vyas A, Whittaker VJ, et al. Dietary advice for treatment of type 2 diabetes mellitus in adults. Cochrane Database Syst Rev 2007;3:1–73.

Norris SL, Zhang X, Avenell A, Gregg E, Schmid CH, Lau J. Long-term non-pharmacological weight loss interventions for adults with prediabetes. Cochrane Database Syst Rev 2005;2:CD005270.

Odegaard AO, Koh W-P, Butler LM, Duval S, Gross MD, Yu MC, et al. Dietary patterns and incident type 2 diabetes in Chinese men and women. The Singapore Chinese Health Study. Diabetes Care 2011;34:880–5.

Onkamo P, Vaananen S, Karvonen M, Tuomilehto J. Worldwide increase in incidence of type I diabetes—the analysis of the data on published incidence trends. Diabetologia 2000;42:1395–403.

Pakenham-Walsh N, Bukachi F. Information needs of health care workers in developing countries: a literature review with a focus on Africa. Hum Resour Health 2009;7:30.

Pasquale LR, Kang JH, Manson JE, Willett WC, Rosner BA, Hankinson SE. Prospective study of type 2 diabetes mellitus and risk of primary open-angle glaucoma in women. Ophthalmology 2006;113:1081–6.

Paterson BL, Charlton P, Richard S. Non-attendance in chronic disease clinics: a matter of non-compliance? J Nurs Health Chronic Illn 2010;2:63–74.

Patterson CC, Dahlquist GG, Gyurus E, Green A, Soltesz G. Incidence trends for childhood type 1 diabetes in Europe during 1989–2003 and predicted new cases 2005–20: a multicentre prospective registration study. Lancet 2009;373:2027–33.

Patton SR. Adherence to diet in youth with type 1 diabetes. J Am Diet Assoc 2011;111:550–5.

Pavkov ME, Burrows NR, Knowler WC, Hanson RI, Neslon RG. Diabetes and chronic kidney disease. In: Narayan KMV, Williams D, Gregg EW, Cowie CC, editors. Diabetes public health. From data to policy. USA: Oxford University Press; 2011.

Perlmuter LC, Flanagan BP, Shah PH, Singh SP. Glycemic control and hypoglycemia. Is the loser the winner? Diabetes Care 2008;31:2072–6.

Pierce M, Agarwal G, Ridout D. A survey of diabetes care in general practice in England and Wales. Br J Gen Pract 2000;50:542–5.

Pollock RD, Unwin NC, Connolly V. Knowledge and practice of foot care in people with diabetes. Diabetes Res Clin Pract 2004;64:117–22.

Popkin BM. Global nutrition dynamics: the world is shifting rapidly toward a diet linked with noncommunicable diseases. Am J Clin Nutr 2006;84:289–98.

Reece EA, Leguizamon G, Wiznitzer A. Gestational diabetes: the need for a common ground. Lancet 2009;373:1789–97.

Resnikoff S, Pascolini D, Etya'ale D, Kocur I, Pararajasegaram R, Pokharel GP, et al. Global data on visual impairment in the year 2002. Bull World Health Organ 2004;82:844.

Rhee MK, Slocum W, Ziemer DC, Culler SD, Cook CB, El-Kebbi IM, et al. Patient adherence improves glycemic control. Diabetes Educ 2005;31:240–50.

Ricco-Cabelli I, Ruiz-Perez I, Olry de Labry-Lima A, Marquez-Calderon S. Do social inequalities exist in terms of the prevention, diagnosis, treatment, control and monitoring of diabetes? A systematic review. Health Soc Care Community 2010;18:572–87.

Roglic G, Unwin N. Mortality attributable to diabetes: estimates for the year 2010. Diab Res Clin Pract 2010;87:15–9.

Ruigomez A, Garcia-Rodriguez LA. Presence of diabetes related complication at the time of NIDDM diagnosis: an important prognostic factor. Eur J Epidemiol 1998;14:439–45.

Safford MM, Russell L, Suh D-C, Roman S, Pogach L. How much time do patients with diabetes spend on self-care? Diabetes Care 2005;18:262–70.

Saydah SH, Eberhardt MS. Diabetes and mortality. In: Narayan KMV, Williams D, Gregg EW, Cowie CC, editors. Diabetes public health. From data to policy. USA: Oxford University Press; 2011.

Schwartz AV, Vitthinghoff E, Sellmeyer DE, Feingold KR, de Rekeneire N, Strotmeyer ES, et al. Diabetes-related complications, glycemic control, and falls in older adults. J Diabetes Complications 2008;31:391–6.

Scottish Diabetes Survey Monitoring Group. Scottish diabetes survey 2013; 2013. http://www.diabetesinscotland.org.uk/Publications/SDS2013.pdf.

Scottish Executive Health Department. Promoting the development of managed clinical networks in NHS Scotland; 2002. NHS Circular: HDL (2002) 69. www.sehd.scot.nhs.uk/mels/HDL2002_69.pdf.

Scottish Intercollegiate Guidelines Network. 116. Management of diabetes. A national clinical guideline; 2010. http://www.sign.ac.uk/pdf/sign116.pdf.

Scottish Government. Obesity route map - action plan; 2011. http://www.gov.scot/Resource/Doc/346007/0115166.pdf.

References

Selvin E, Burnett AL, Platz EA. Prevalence and risk factors for erectile dysfunction in the US. Am Med J 2007;120:151–7.

Shaw S, Rosen R, Rumbold B. What is integrated care? The Nuffield Trust; 2011. http://www.nuffieldtrust. org.uk/sites/files/nuffield/publication/what_is_ integrated_care_research_report_june11_0.pdf.

Simmons RK, Coleman RL, Price HC, Holman RR, Khaw K-T, Wareham NJ, et al. Performance of the UK Prospective Diabetes Study Risk Engine and the Framingham Risk Equations in estimating cardiovascular disease in the EPIC- Norfolk Cohort. Diabetes Care 2009;32:708–13.

Simmons RK, Echouffo-Tcheugui JB, Sharp SJ, Sargeant LA, Williams KM, Prevost AT, et al. Screening for type 2 diabetes and population mortality over 10 years (ADDITION-Cambridge): a cluster-randomised controlled trial. Lancet 2012;380:1741–8.

Sinclair AJ, Conroy SP, Bayer AJ. Impact of diabetes on physical function in older people. Diabetes Care 2008;31:233–5.

Singh N, Armstrong DG, Lipsky BA. Preventing foot ulcers in patients with diabetes. Clin Rev 2005;293:217–28.

Smith DB. Urinary incontinence and diabetes: a review. J Wound Ostomy Continence Nurs 2006;33:619–23.

Smith-Spangler CM, Bhattacharya J, Goldhaber-Fiebert JD. Diabetes, its treatment, and catastrophic medical spending in 35 developing countries. Diabetes Care 2012;35:319–26.

Snow R, Fulop N. Understanding issues associated with attending a young adult diabetes clinic: a case study. Diabet Med 2012;29:257–9.

Soedamah-Muthu SS, Fuller JH, Mulnier HE, Raleigh VS, Lawrenson RA, Colhoun HM. High risk of cardiovascular disease in patients with type 1 diabetes in the U.K.: a cohort study using the general practice research database. Diabetologia 2006;29:798–804.

Spijkerman AM, Henry RM, Dekker JM, Nijpels G, Kostense PJ, Kors JA, et al. Prevalence of macrovascular disease amongst type 2 diabetic patients detected by targeted screening and patients newly diagnosed in general practice: the Hoorn Screening Study. J Intern Med 2004;256:429–36.

Stockwell T, Zhao J, Giesbrecht N, Macdonald S, Thomas G, Wettlaufer A. The raising of minimum alcohol prices in Saskatchewan, Canada: impacts on consumption and implications for public health. Am J Public Health 2012;102:e103–10. http://ajph.aphapublications.org/doi/abs/10.2105/ AJPH.2012.301094.

The Action to Control Cardiovascular Risk in Diabetes Study Group. Effects of intensive glucose lowering in type 2 diabetes. N Engl J Med 2008;358:2545–9.

The DECODE Study Group. Age- and sex-specific prevalences of diabetes and impaired glucose regulation in 13 European cohorts. Diabetes Care 2003;26:61–9.

The Diabetes Control and Complications Trial/ Epidemiology of Diabetes Interventions and Complications (DCCT/EDIC) Study Research Group. Intensive diabetes treatment and cardiovascular disease in patients with type 1 diabetes. N Engl J Med 2005;353:2643–53.

The Emerging Risk Factors Collaboration. The Emerging Risk Factors Collaboration: analysis of individual data on lipid, inflammatory and other markers in over 1.1 million participants in 104 prospective studies of cardiovascular diseases. Eur J Epidemiol 2007;22:839–69.

The Emerging Risk Factors Collaboration. Diabetes mellitus, fasting blood glucose concentration, and risk of vascular disease: a collaborative meta-analysis of 102 prospective studies. Lancet 2010;375:2215–22.

The NHS Information Centre. National diabetes audit executive summary; 2011.

The Information Centre. Health survey for England 2006; 2008. www.ic.nhs.uk/webfiles/publications/ HSE06/HSE%2006%20report%20VOL%20 1%20v2.pdf.

The Information Centre. National diabetes audit executive summary 2009–2010; 2011. http://www. hqip.org.uk/assets/NCAPOP-Library/National-Diabetes-Audit-Executive-Summary-2009-2010.pdf.

Thomason MJ, Biddulph JP, Cull CA, Holman RR. Reporting of death on death certificates using data from the UK Prospective Diabetes Study. Diabet Med 2005;22:1031–6.

Tuomilehto J, Lindström J, Eriksson JG, Valle TT, Hämäläinen H, Ilanne-Parikka P, et al. Prevention of type 2 diabetes mellitus by changes in lifestyle among subjects with impaired glucose tolerance. N Engl J Med 2001;344:1343–50.

United Kingdom Prospective Diabetes Study Group. Complications in newly diagnosed type 2 diabetic patients and their association with different clinical and biochemical risk factors (UKPDS VI). Diabetes Res 1990;13:1–11.

United Kingdom Prospective Diabetes Study Group. Intensive blood-glucose control with sulphonylureas or insulin compared with conventional treatment and risk of complications in patients with type 2 diabetes (UKPDS 33). Lancet 1998a;352:837–53.

United Kingdom Prospective Diabetes Study Group. Tight blood pressure control and risk of macrovascular and microvascular complications in type 2 diabetes: UKPDS 38. Br Med J 1998b;317:703–13.

Valk GD, Kriegsman DM, Assendelft WJ. Patient education for preventing diabetic foot ulceration. Cochrane Database Syst Rev 2001;4:CD001488.

Venkataraman K, Kannan AT, Mohan V. Challenges in diabetes management with particular reference to India. Int J Diabetes Dev Ctries 2009;29:103–9.

Vermeire EIJJ, Wens J, van Royen P, Biot Y, Hearnshaw H, Lindenmeyer A. Interventions for improving adherence to treatment recommendations in people with type 2 diabetes mellitus. Cochrane Metabolic and Endocrine Disorders Group; 2009. Doi: 10.1002/14651858.CD003638.pub2.

Volpato S, Maraldi C. Diabetes and disability, cognitive decline and aging-related outcomes. In: Narayan KMV, Williams D, Gregg EW, Cowie CC, editors. Diabetes public health. From data to policy. USA: Oxford University Press; 2011.

Wanatabe RM, Black MH, Xiang AH, Allayee H, Lawrence JM, Buchanan TA. Genetics of gestational diabetes mellitus and type 2 diabetes. Diabetes Care 2007;30:S134–40.

Waugh N, Scotland G, McNamee P, Gillett M, Brennan A, Goyder E, et al. Screening for type 2 diabetes: literature review and economic modelling. Health Technol Assess 2007;11:17.

WHO/IDF Consultation Group. Definition and diagnosis of diabetes mellitus and intermediate hyperglycaemia: report of a WHO/IDF consultation. Geneva: World Health Organization; 2006.

Wild S. Relative risk of mortality associated with diabetes in Scotland in 2007: a nationwide record linkage study. J Epidemiol Community Health 2009;63:62.

Wild S, Roglic G, Green A, Sicree R, King H. Global prevalence of diabetes. Estimates for the year 2000 and projections for 2030. Diabetes Care 2004;27:1047–53.

Williams R, Airey M, Baxter H, Forrester J, Kennedy-Martin T, Girach A. Epidemiology of diabetic retinopathy and macular oedema: a systematic review. Eye 2004;18:963–83.

Wilson JMG, Jungner G. Principles and practice of screening for disease. Geneva: World Health Organization; 1968.

Woolthius EPK, de Grauw WJC, van Gerwen WHEM, van den Hoogen HJM, van de Lisdonk EM, Metsemakers JFM, et al. Yield of opportunistic targeted screening for type 2 diabetes in primary care: the Diabscreen study. Ann Fam Med 2009;7:422–30.

World Health Organization. Definition, diagnosis and classification of diabetes mellitus and its complications. Report of a WHO Consultation. Part 1: diagnosis and classification of diabetes mellitus. Geneva: World Health Organization; 1999.

World Health Organization. Adherence to long-term therapies: evidence for action; 2003a.

World Health Organization. Screening for type 2 diabetes. Report of a World Health Organization and International Diabetes Federation meeting; 2003b.

World Health Organization. The global burden of disease: 2004 update. Geneva: World Health Organization; 2008.

World Health Organization. Global status report on noncommunicable diseases. Geneva: World Health Organization; 2010.

World Health Organization. Diabetes fact sheet No. 312 August 2011; 2011a. http://www.who.int/mediacentre/factsheets/fs312/en/index.html (accessed 17.07.12).

World Health Organization. Use of glycated haemoglobin (HbA1c) in the diagnosis of diabetes mellitus. Abbreviated report of a WHO Consultation. Geneva: World Health Organization; 2011a.

World Health Organization. WHO list of essential medicines; 2011b. http://whqlibdoc.who.int/hq/2011/a95053_eng.pdf.

World Health Organization, Diabetes Fact Sheet. No. 312; 2015. http://www.who.int/mediacentre/factsheets/fs312/en/.

Yach D, Stuckler D, Brownell K. Epidemiologic and economic consequences of the global epidemics of obesity and diabetes. Nat Med 2006;12:62–6.

Yates T, Davies MJ, Sehmi S, Gorely T, Khunit K. The Pre-diabetes Risk Education and Physical Activity Recommendation and Encouragement (PREPARE) programme study: are improvements in glucose regulation sustained at 2 years? Diabet Med 2011;10:1268–71.

YHPHO. Yorkshire and Humberside Public Health Authority. Diabetes Attributable Deaths: Estimating the excess deaths among people with diabetes; 2008. http://www.yhpho.org.uk/resource/item.aspx?RID=9909.

Zhang X, Brown J, Vistisen D, Sicree R, Shaw J, Nichols G. Global healthcare expenditure on diabetes for 2010 and 2030. Diabetes Res Clin Pract 2010;87:293–301.

Index

Note: Page numbers followed by *f* indicate figures, *b* indicate boxes and *t* indicate tables.

Index

Index